2/10

marie claire GORGEOUS FACE & BEAUTIFUL BODY

JOSETTE MILGRAM
TRANSLATED BY
KIM ALLEN GLEED

marie claire GORGEOUS FACE & BEAUTIFUL BODY

A GUIDE TO TOTAL SKIN CARE

HEARST BOOKS
A division of Sterling Publishing Co., Inc.

New York / London
www.sterlingpublishing.com

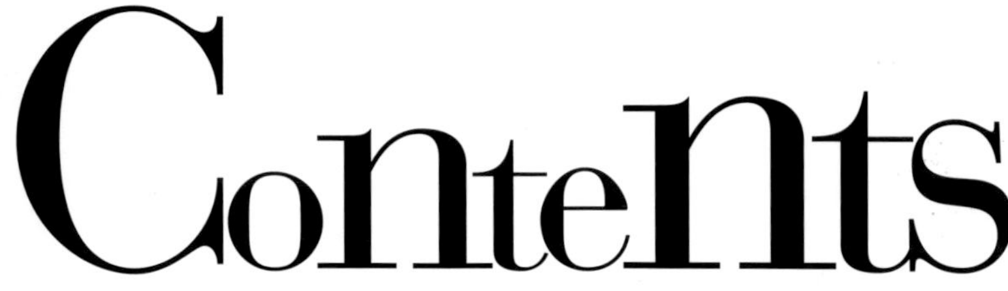

MAKE YOUR BEAUTY DREAMS COME TRUE

1. At the heart of your skin

BEAUTY ESSENTIALS

2. At the heart of your body

IMPORTANT POINTS

3. Skin & body care: favorite treatments

SKIN CARE: IN-YOUR-FACE BEAUTY

BODY CARE: PERFECT HARMONY

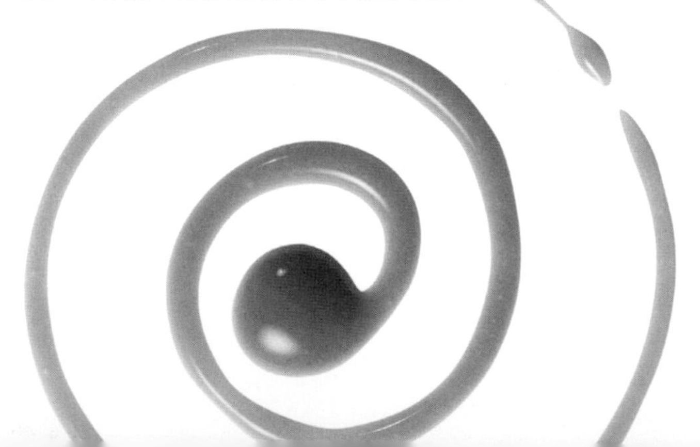

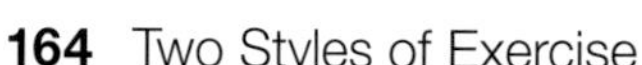

4. Balance YOUR FIGURE

TAKE A BITE OUT OF LIFE BY ENJOYING HEALTHY FOODS

5. Anti-aging TAMING TIME

6. Well-being EVERYDAY ROUTINES

7. Amazing You THE BEST IN THE WORLD

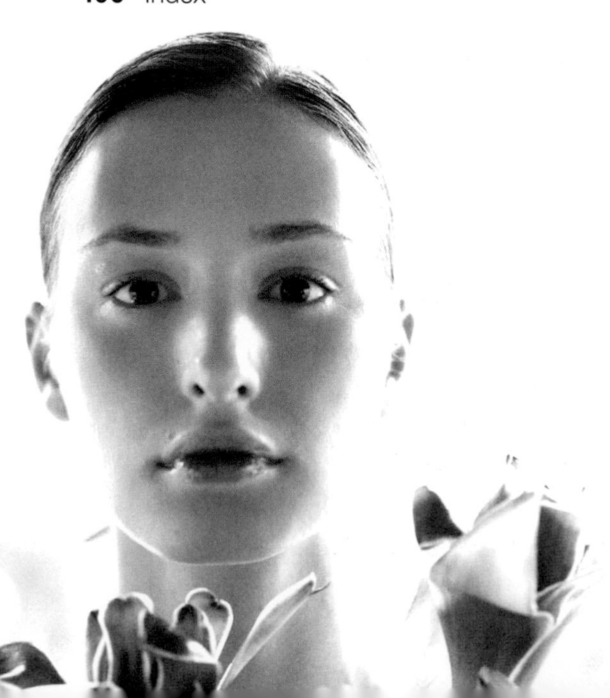

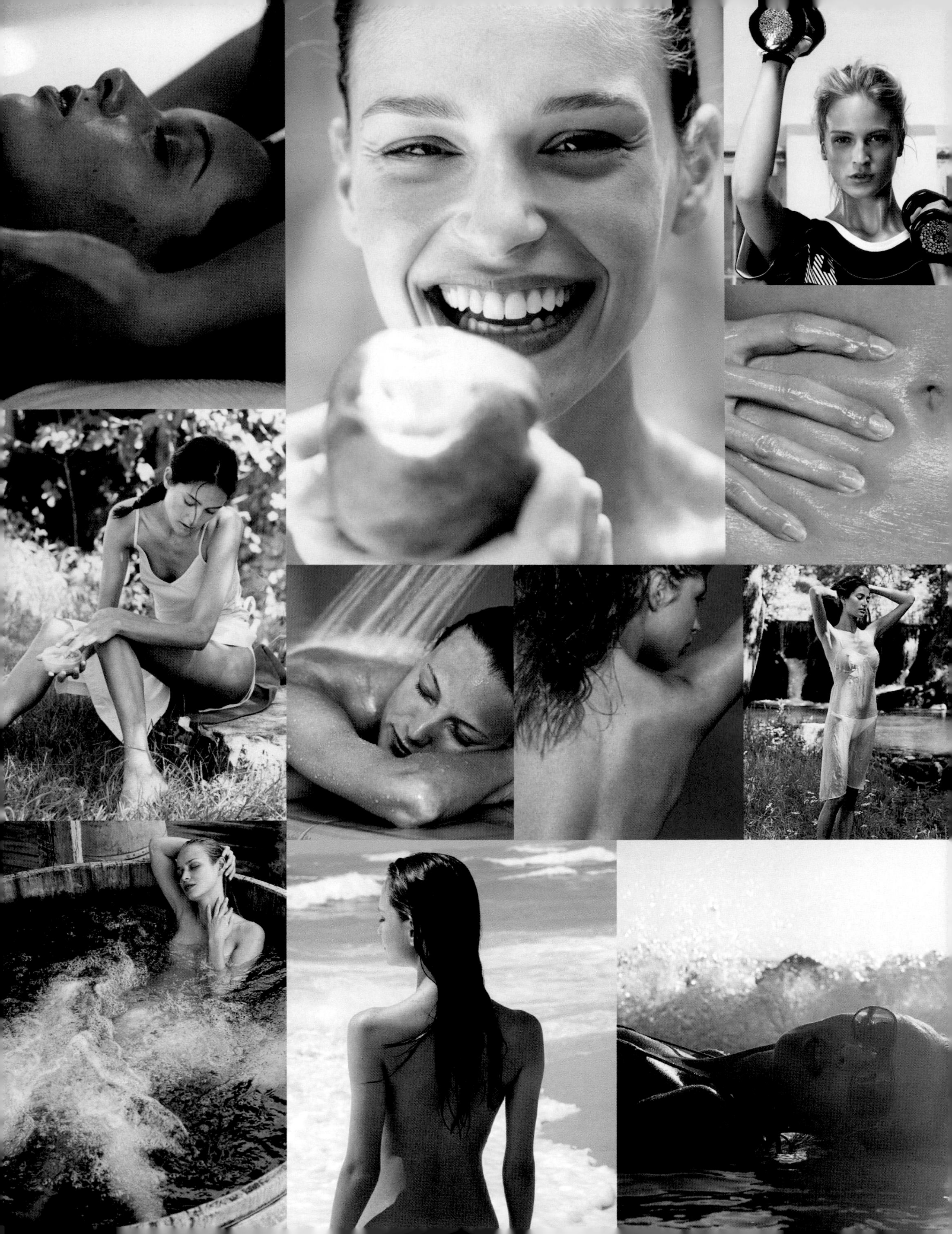

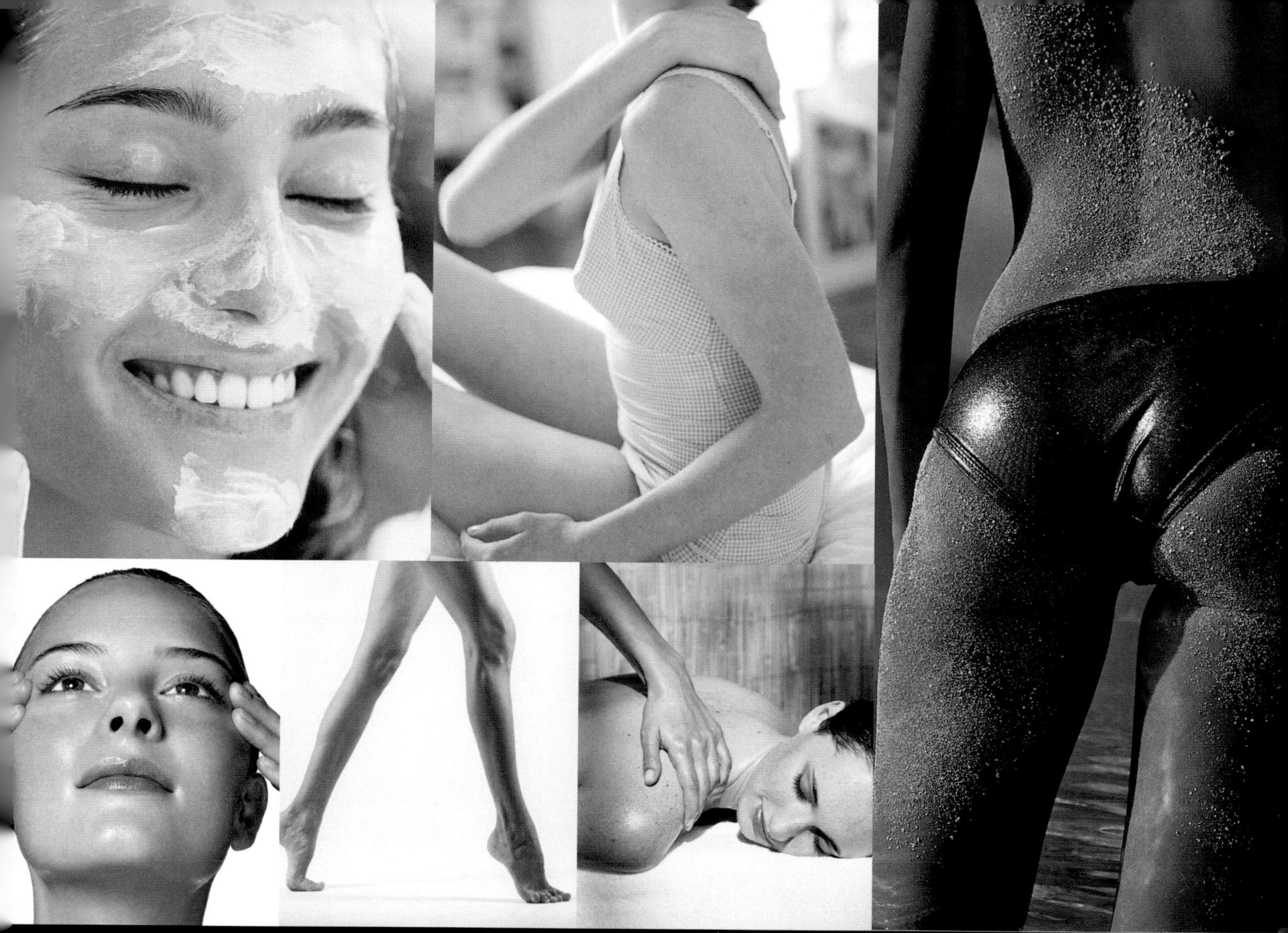

Make your beauty dreams come true.

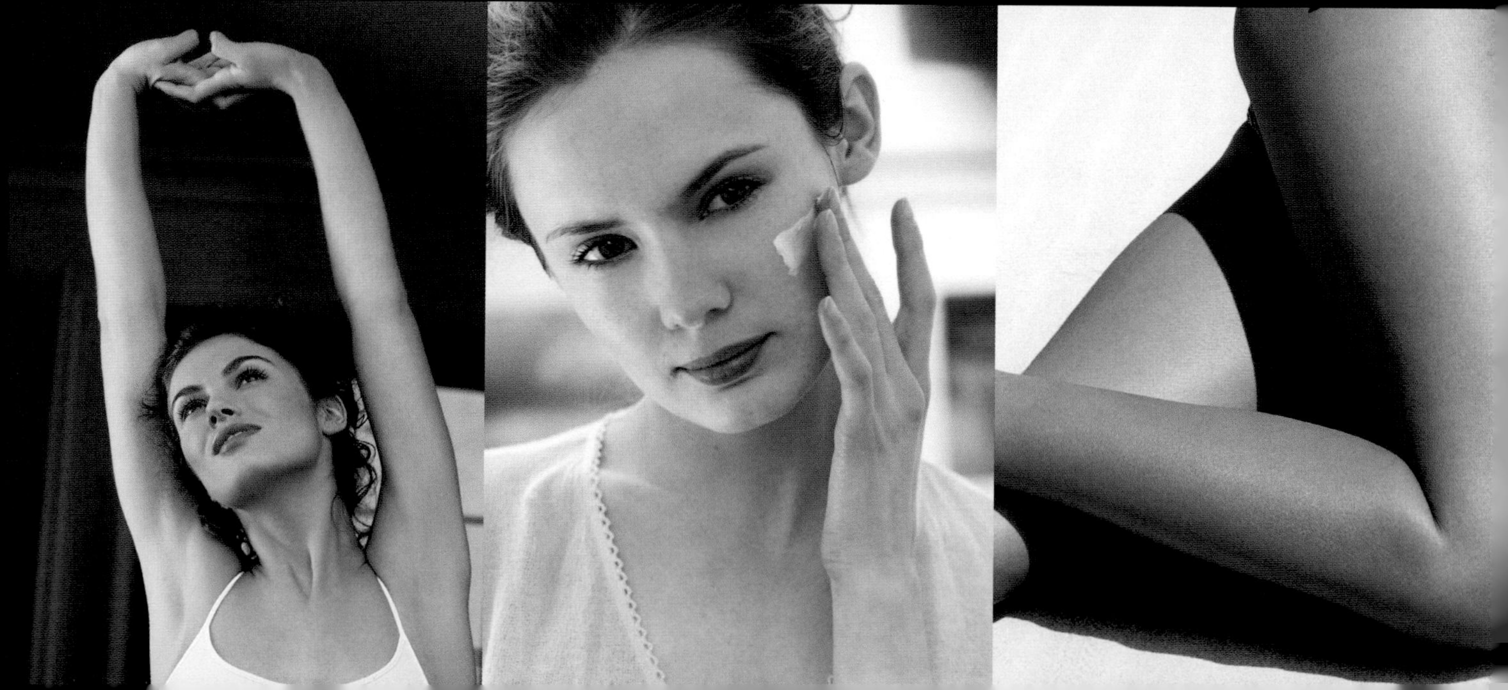

1

at the heart of your skin

BEAUTY ESSENTIALS

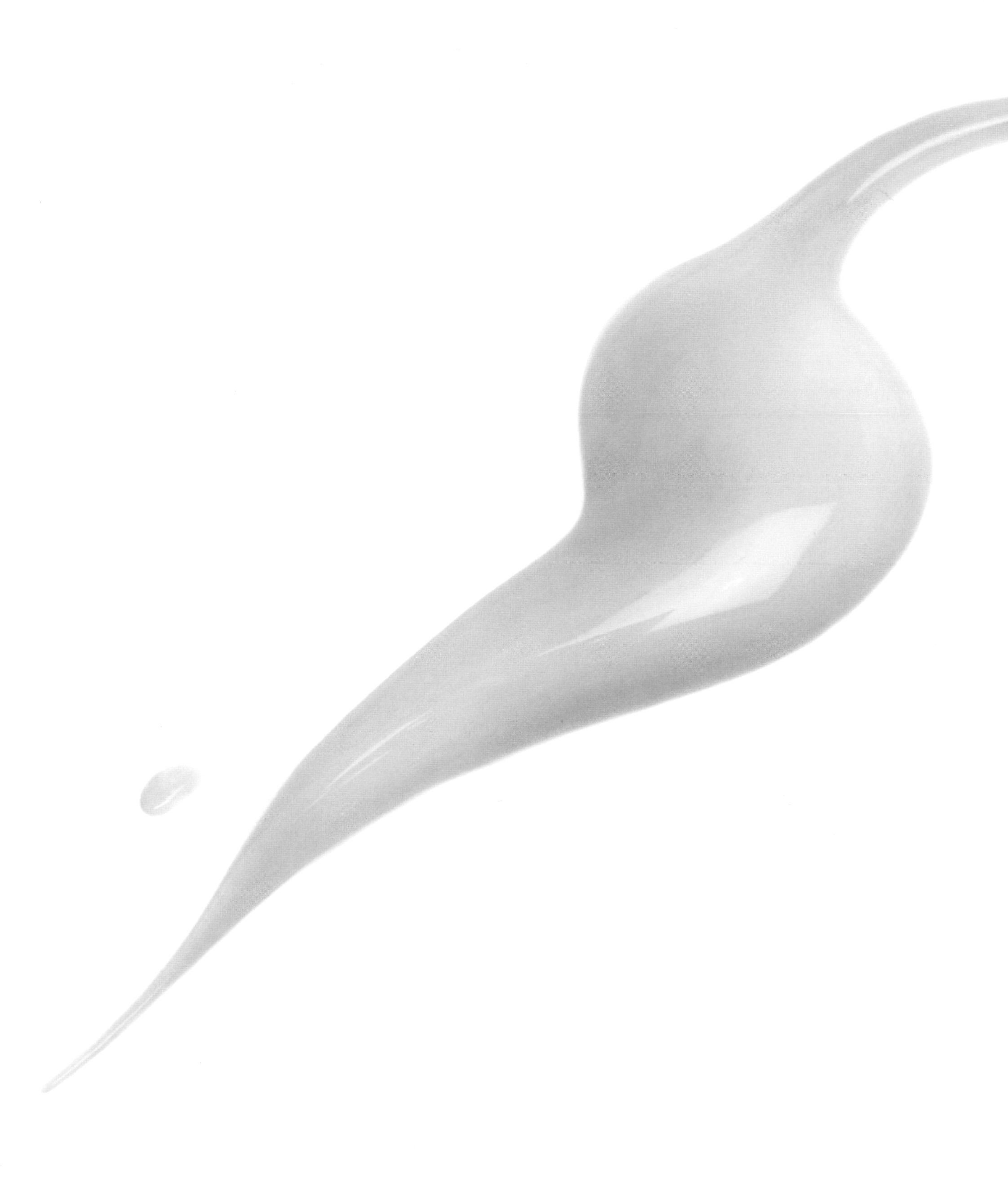

BEAUTY ESSENTIALS

The reflection of your being starts at the surface with your skin

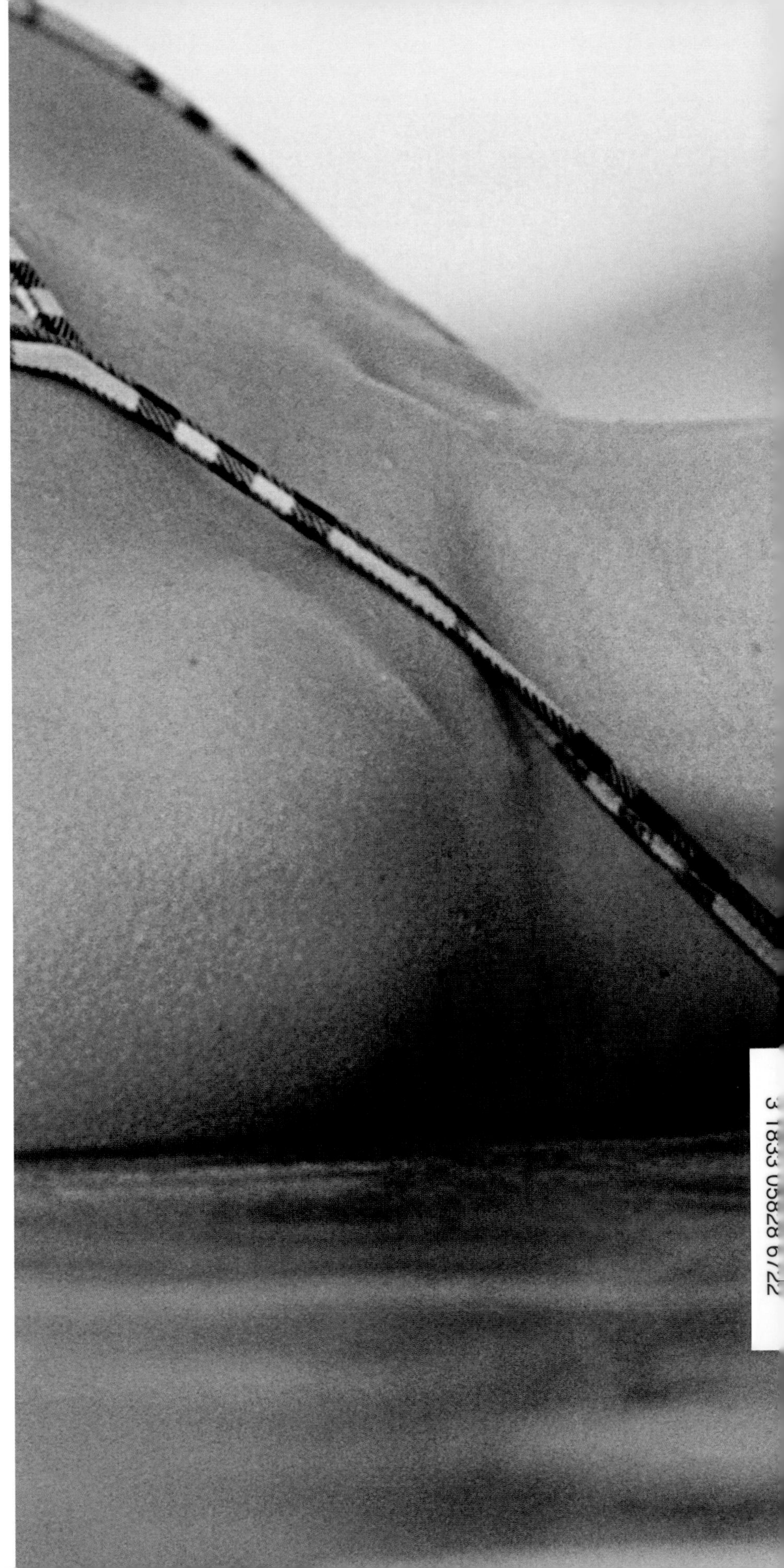

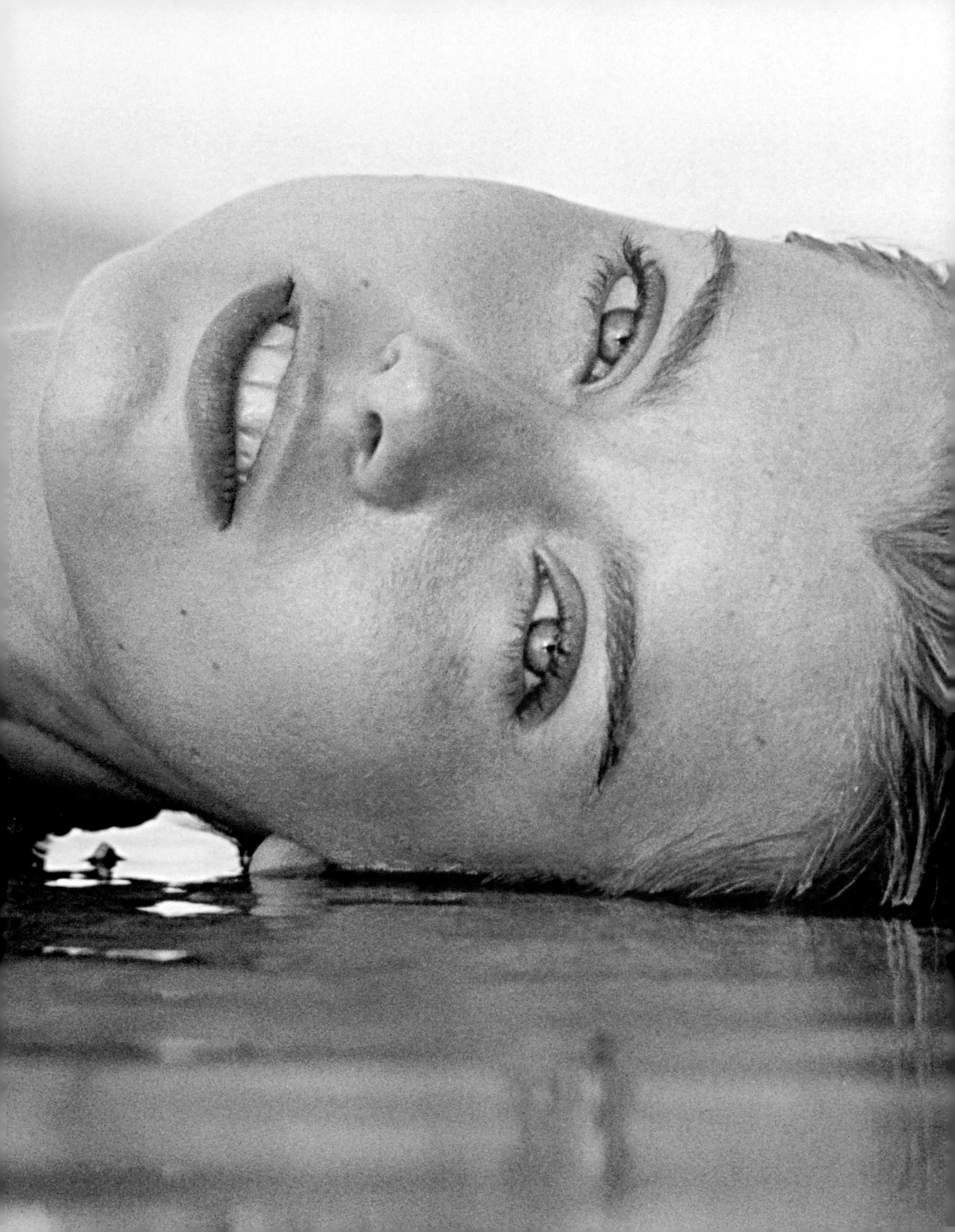

The secret life of skin

The largest organ of your body, skin is the most effective cover for survival. Its incredible features deserve an in-depth, guided tour.

Skin can protect... Cutaneous receptors instantly transmit to our brain all sorts of information. They tell us if something is soft, hot, sharp, etc. **And skin can heal...** Absorbing oxygen and emitting carbon dioxide, skin diffuses these important elements in blood. • The proof of collagen's resiliency? It's what remains when animal skin is turned into leather!

ADVICE FROM A DERMATOLOGIST
Skin's stratum corneum has an average of 5 to 10 layers, but there are 20 layers on the back and hundreds of layers on the soles of the feet. Mucous membranes, however, do not have this layer of skin.

SKIN IS THE MOST INTELLIGENT OF MATERIALS

With an area of nearly 22 square feet ranging from 0.05 to 0.15 inches thick and weighing approximately 6.5 pounds, in terms of volume, skin is **our largest vital organ.** A unique combination of 2 trillion hyperactive cells, it ensures the protection of our entire physical being. Skin analyzes everything in our environment to regulate our temperature, keeping us from becoming too hot or too cold. It also forms a barrier against ultraviolet rays, destroys harmful bacteria, and generates antibodies. A vital interface with the outside world, skin has **three layers of high protection.**

THE EPIDERMIS

From a thickness of only 0.002 inches on the eyelids to 0.8 to 0.12 inches on the soles of the feet, the epidermis is the layer of skin that is in direct contact with the outside world. Its mission: to prevent all intruders from penetrating our skin. Its exceptional longevity is the result of the perpetual renewal of cells called **keratinocytes,** which continually migrate from the **basal layer** (the boundary between the epidermis and the dermis) toward the surface, where they stack into little piles to become **corneocytes.** They take 28 days to "ripen," developing into a shell that makes up the **corneal layer (stratum corneum),** before drying out and flaking off to make room for future generations. The **hydrolipidic film,** a blend of perspiration and sebum (oil), guarantees the balance of water in our skin. If this protective layer is disturbed, the corneal layer, which is much less hydrated, will thicken and age prematurely. ▶

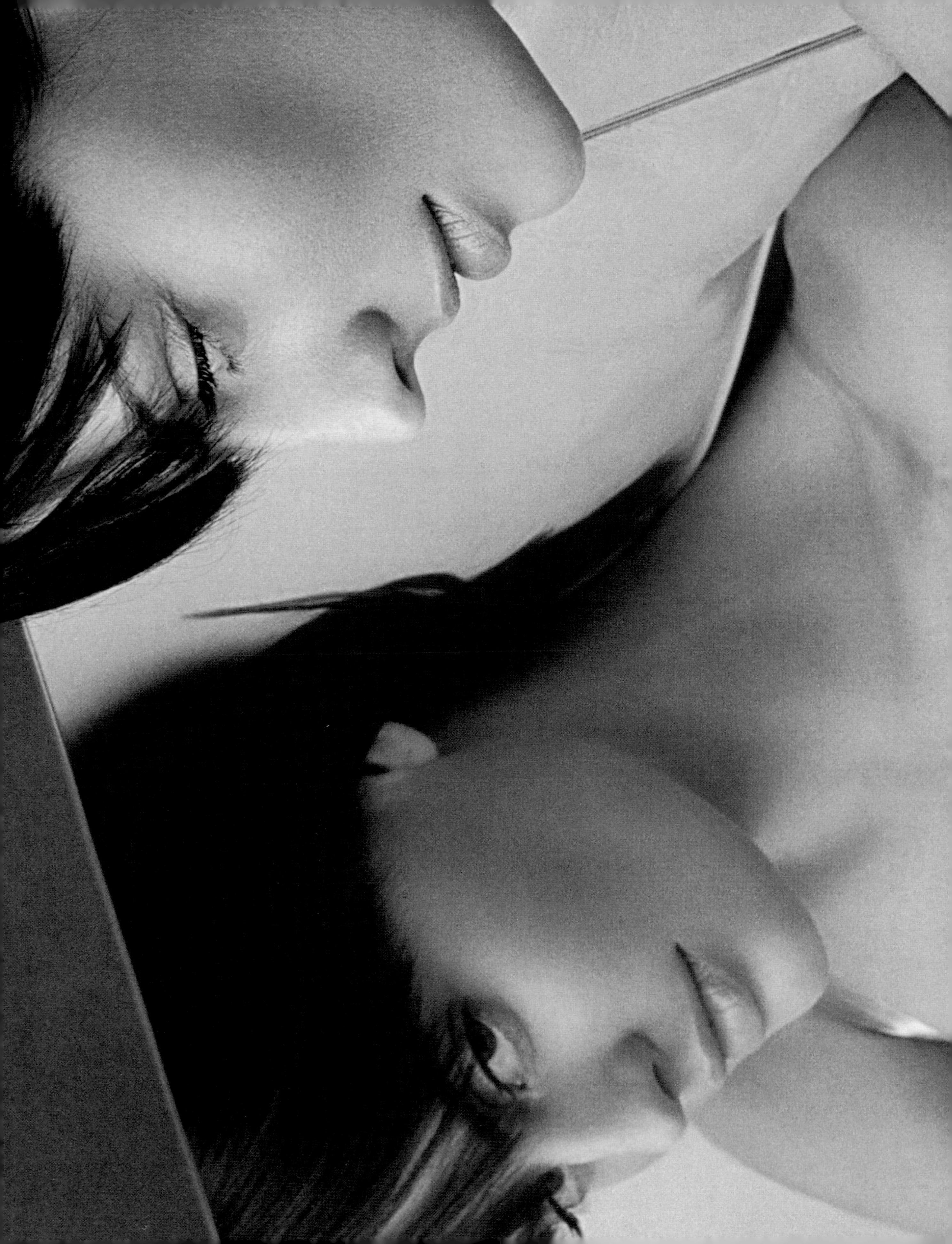

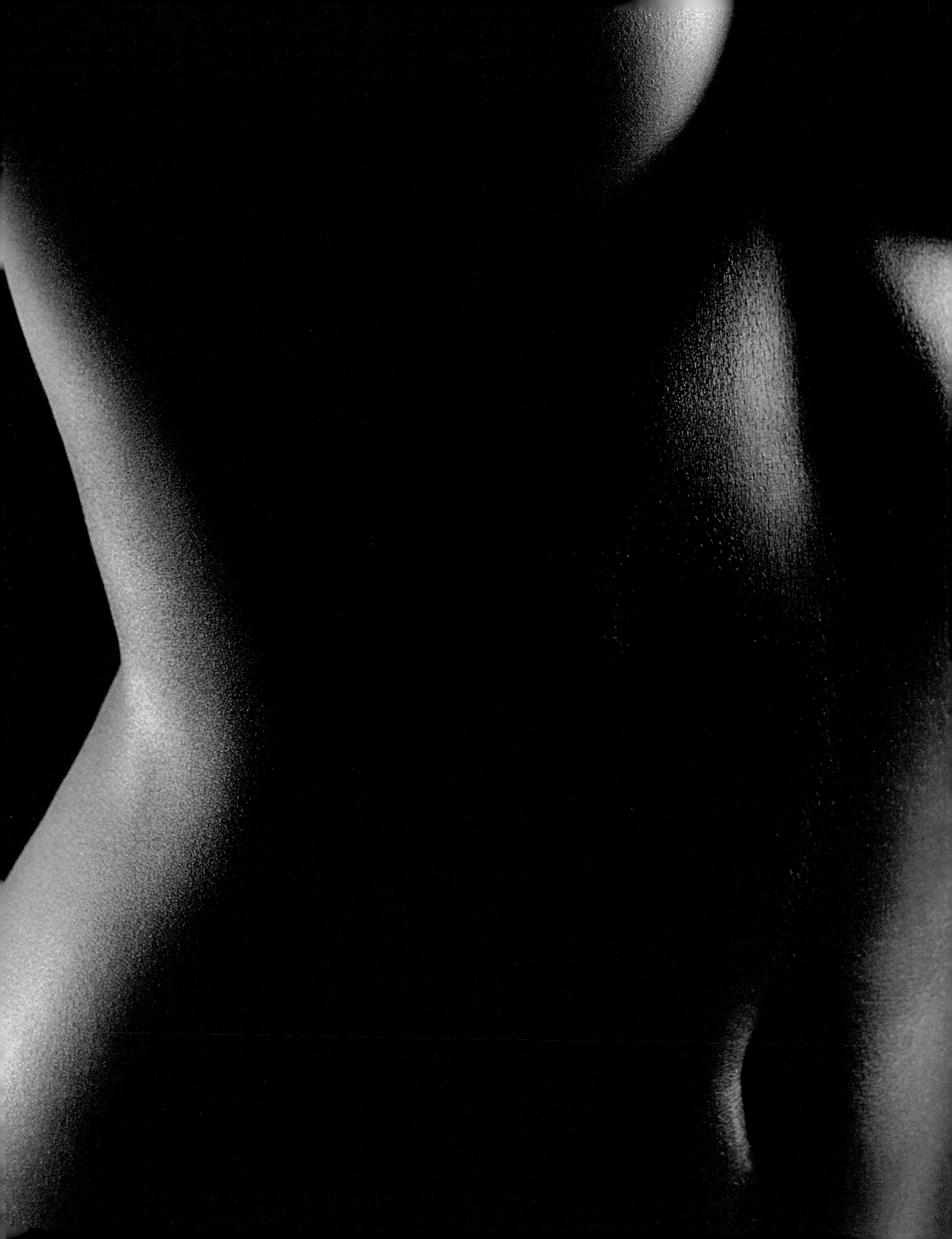

▶ THE DERMIS

This is the thickest layer of skin, and it is both solid and supple. This supporting tissue, which bears the epidermis, gives skin its consistency, elasticity, and tone. The cells in the dermis (**fibroblasts**) produce proteins that allow the regulation of water: the **collagen** fibers ensure solidity, and **elastin** gives skin the ability to assume its normal shape again after being stretched. When it comes to the signs of skin aging, it's the dermis we're talking about! It is crisscrossed by nourishing blood vessels that feed the epidermis, and a countless number of nerves that faithfully report to the brain every unfortunate event felt by their sensors. They transmit instructions when they feel heat (causing us to perspire), cold (causing the vessels to contract and turn our skin pale), or pain (causing us to shriek!).

THE HYPODERMIS

The shock absorber and "pantry" of the skin, this layer is full of lipids. Situated below the dermis, the hypodermis has the primary function of stockpiling reserves that we can use when there is a shortage of food or energy. It also protects us from cold. The cells that allow us to store fats, **adipocytes,** are dispersed differently according to sex: while they prefer to make their home in the stomach area for men, in women they have a predilection for thighs and buttocks—this is what causes pear-shaped silhouettes! The unfortunate visible result when accumulated fats and water are trapped in the tissue? Cellulite.

Our dermis is composed of 70 percent water. Skin contains 25 to 35 percent of all the water reserves in our body, approximately 2.5 gallons.

ADVICE FROM A DOCTOR

Men have (almost) no cellulite. Women's fatty tissue represents 23 percent of body weight as opposed to only 15 percent for men. The explanation for this genetic injustice? Women are programmed to ensure the survival of the species!

Your Skin's True Nature: A Quick Diagnostic

A verdict you cannot appeal: your skin will evolve and change ajust as you do! It will glow when everything is going well and cry for help when you are under stress. You must listen to it.

The ideal level of hydration for the stratum corneum is 13%. If it falls to 10% or below, skin is dry.

The oily power of the sebaceous glands protects us from bacteria. And sebum, working in collaboration with water, makes up the very important hydrolipidic film.

ADVICE FROM A DOCTOR

Avoid wearing clothing that is too tight on your body because it blocks the circulation of blood and lymphatic vessels, causing pockets of cellulite and varicose veins, thus altering the texture of your skin. How do you know if your clothes are too tight? When you undress, you should not see any signs of compression!

NORMAL SKIN

A state of grace: almost invisible pores, even tone, natural glow. Preserve this balance!

COMBINATION SKIN

The **T-zone** (forehead, nose, chin), thanks to more active oil glands in this specific area, is shinier than the rest of your face, which might even have dry skin.

OILY SKIN

The only true test: place a piece of tissue paper on your freshly washed face. If there are traces of oil on the paper, you have oily skin. The symptoms: blackheads (clogs due to sebum that is too thick to flow) and pimples, due to the overabundance of oil. Don't be aggressive with this skin type; you must understand its needs and perhaps even get a dermatologist's advice.

DRY SKIN

Dry skin is extremely fragile. The warning sign: if skin feels tight a half hour after washing, the hydrolipidic film is defective, and bacteria can easily gain access. On the body, the most-exposed areas—elbows, knees, and feet—are especially prone to dryness.

SENSITIVE SKIN

Irritable and reactive, sensitive skin seems unable to tolerate anything and makes this known through its coloring, ranging from pink to red; by stinging; and by making all contact unbearable. The good news: this can simply be a transitional phase as a result of pollution or stress. If a product is the sensitivity trigger, you'll be able to determine so with a bit of patience (it takes about two months know if a product is appropriate for your skin).

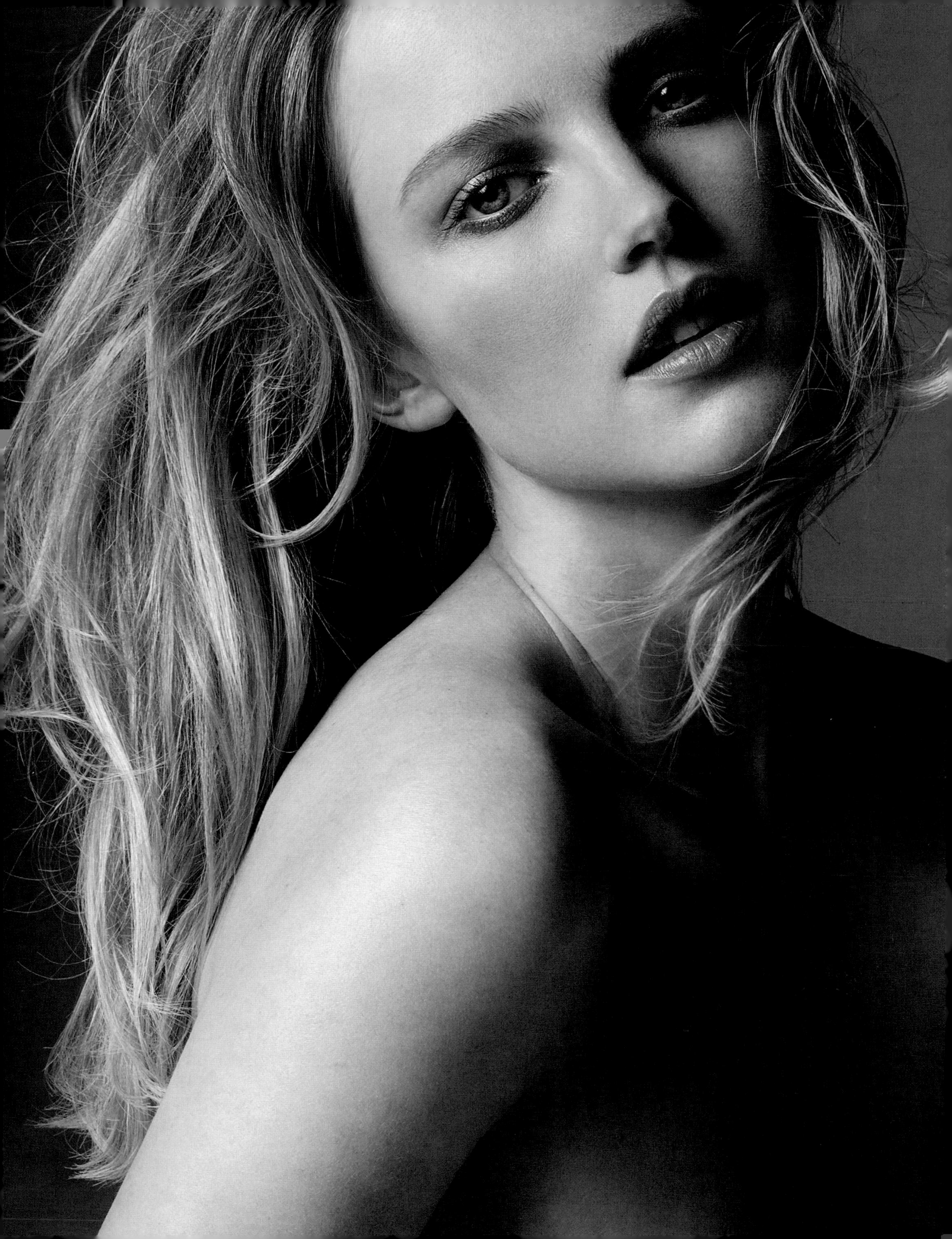

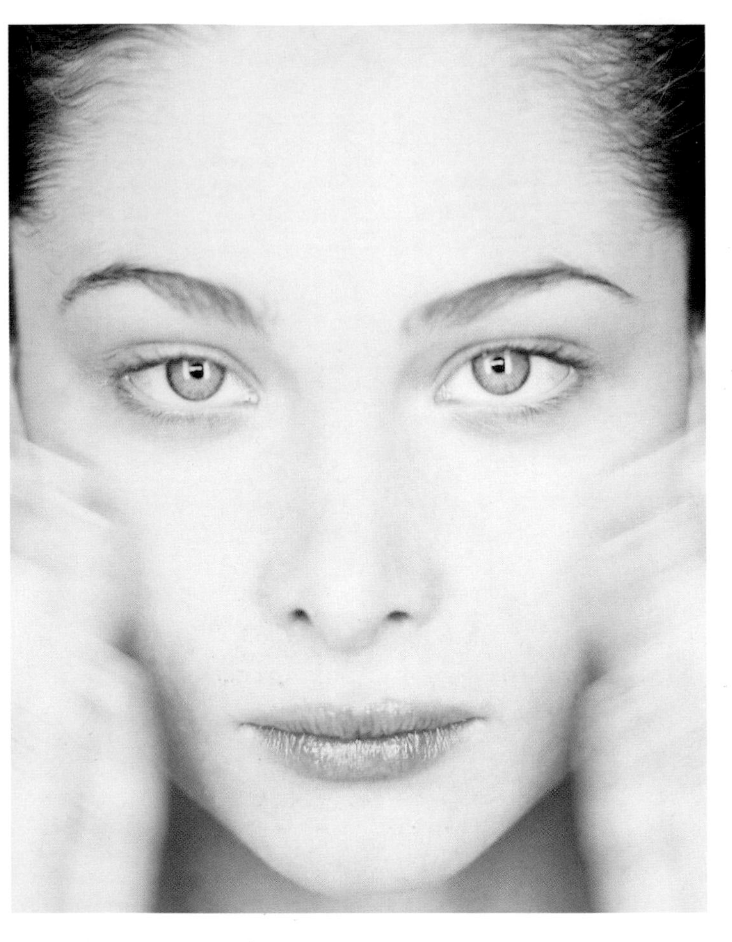
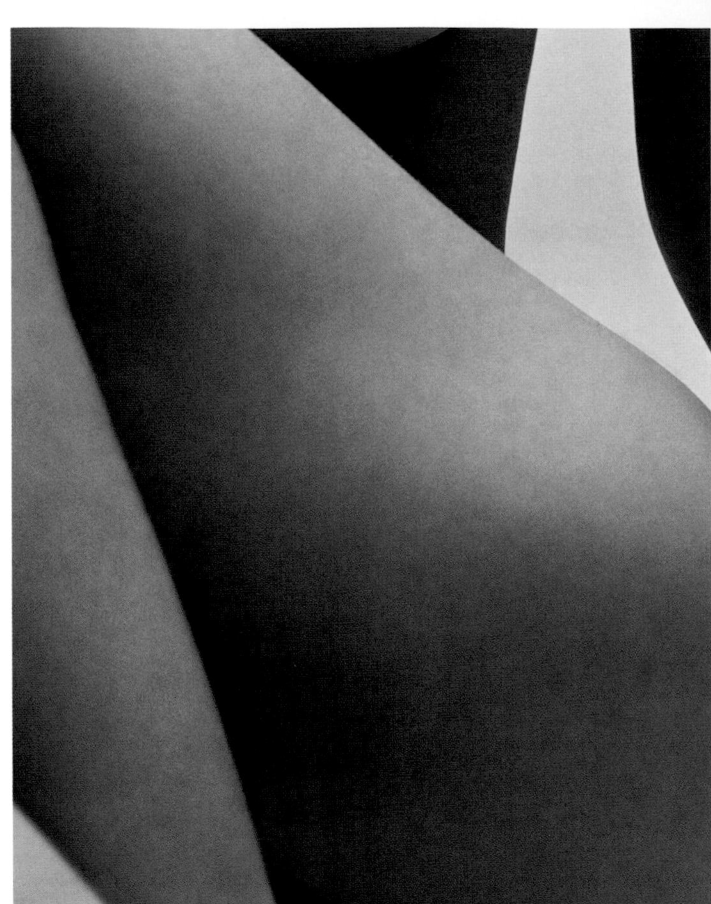
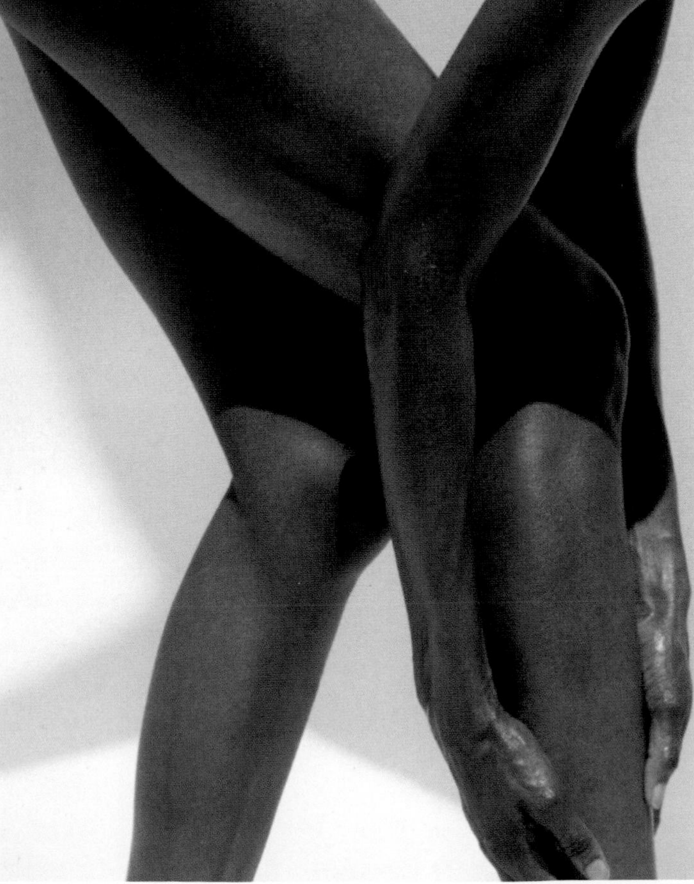
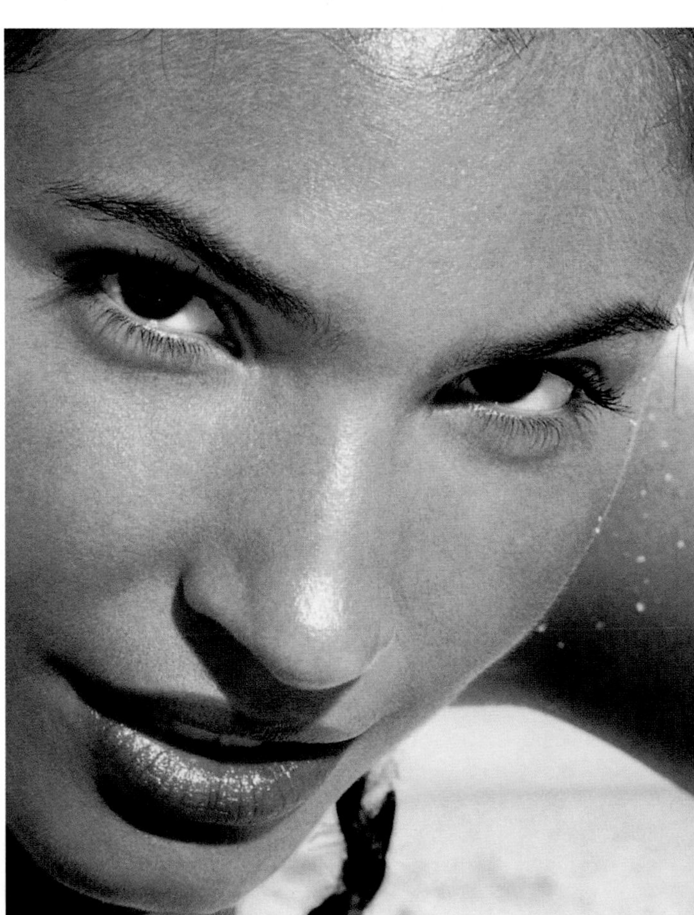

Phototypes: the sun and your skin

We are not all equal in the eyes of the sun: melanin differentiates us in our reactions to UV rays.

OUR EPIDERMIS IS TRANSPARENT!

A pigment called **melanin,** produced by the "suntan" cells called **melanocytes,** tints our skin to protect us from the sun, creating a sort of natural biological parasol otherwise known as **tanning.** The balance between **eumelanin** (the true black melanin) and **pheomelanin** (orange melanin) explains the existence of all the different skin shades under the same sun.

In addition to the **four phototypes** (levels of skin sensitivity to the sun), which range from very light to very dark, scientists also classify us on a scale from one to eight (albino, redhead with milk white skin, golden brown with light skin, blond with light skin, chestnut with light skin, light brown with medium skin, brown with medium skin, black) based on descending risk in relation to M.E.D., minimum erythema dose, or the time of exposure before getting a sunburn. Having this information allows us to reap the benefits of the sun before they are transformed into problems for our skin.

Our reserves of melanin are not only not exhaustible (melanocytes begin to **diminish when we turn 30,** causing us to be less protected against UV rays and increasing our risk for melanoma), but they are also very variable; some people have **three times as many** as others. And if you tan better on certain parts of your body, it's because skin has a memory. The arms, most frequently exposed, are the best trained.

The synthesis of vitamin D, which takes place with the help of ultraviolet light, is critical because it permits the absorption of calcium into the digestive system and promotes its assimilation in bones. (But that doesn't mean you should bake in the sun!)

Melanocytes, which synthesize melanin, have a hefty task: there is only one of them for every 35 keratinocytes.

The epidermis is not a powerful enough parasol: without sunscreen, 30 percent of UVA rays, the ones that age skin, and 10 percent of UVB rays, the ones that burn it (both types can cause skin cancer), are able to reach the dermis.

Beautiful at 20 ...and at every age!

The ideal of eternal beauty is the dream of a modern-day Cleopatra. At the heart of our cells is the future of our skin.

THE AGE OF YOUR SKIN

There is nothing more alive than skin. The dream of taut, baby-soft skin with an unblemished perfection and without any visible pores meets its end when hormones awaken in our teens. At the same time, the production of oily sebum is triggered. The pores open to allow the overabundant sebum to flow, and blackheads and pimples may appear on the epidermis, which has thickened.

Hormones transmit all kinds of information in a network that functions a bit like a biological Internet. Each cell's nucleus, like a hard drive, stores the data.

WHEN TO REVERSE TIME

The synthesis of fibers slows down: skin that is aging sees a degrading of its fibroblasts, the crossbars of skin upon which the blanket of epidermis rests. This combination must be in good shape no matter how old we are! Because our skin type is defined when we are between 15 and 20 years of age, it's wise to anticipate the future: hydrating products are very beneficial in adolescence and have an obvious preventive effect.The **mitochondria** are our central energy factories, transforming the glucose produced in digestion into direct energy used by the cells. They use food to provide 90 percent of the body's energy but also produce the **free radicals** responsible for aging and degenerative illnesses: cellular DNA receives 10,000 attacks from free radicals every day! The list of annoyances resulting from free radicals includes thickening of the stratum corneum, less elasticity, a slowing down of the turnover of cells, reduction in the activity of the melanocytes, and an uneven skin tone. ▶

AT-HOME TEST
Loose skin? To find out, take 10 seconds. Pinch your cheek or the back of your hand, watch, and count. If the fold goes away in less than 10 seconds, no need to worry. If the mark lasts longer, a firming treatment would be beneficial.

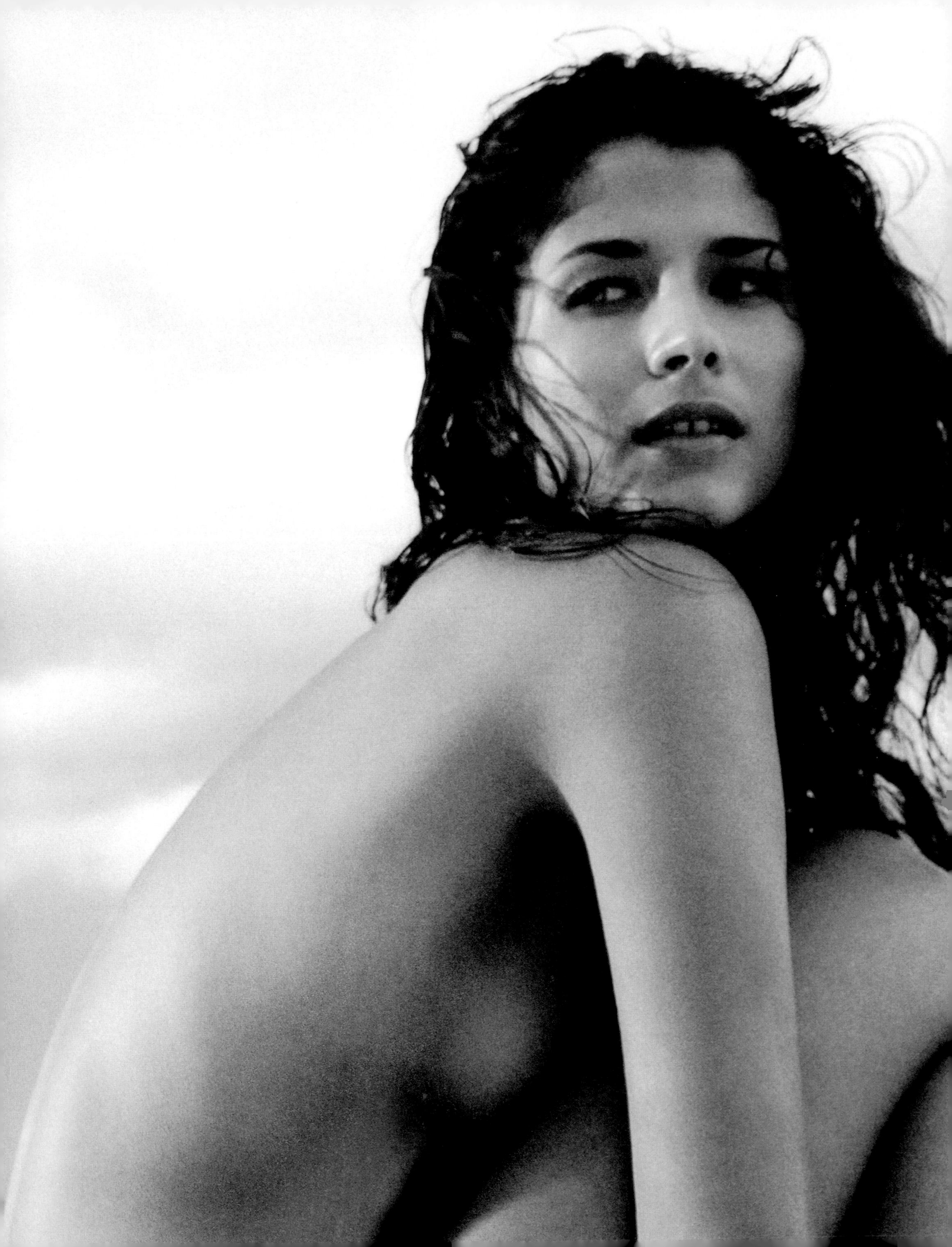

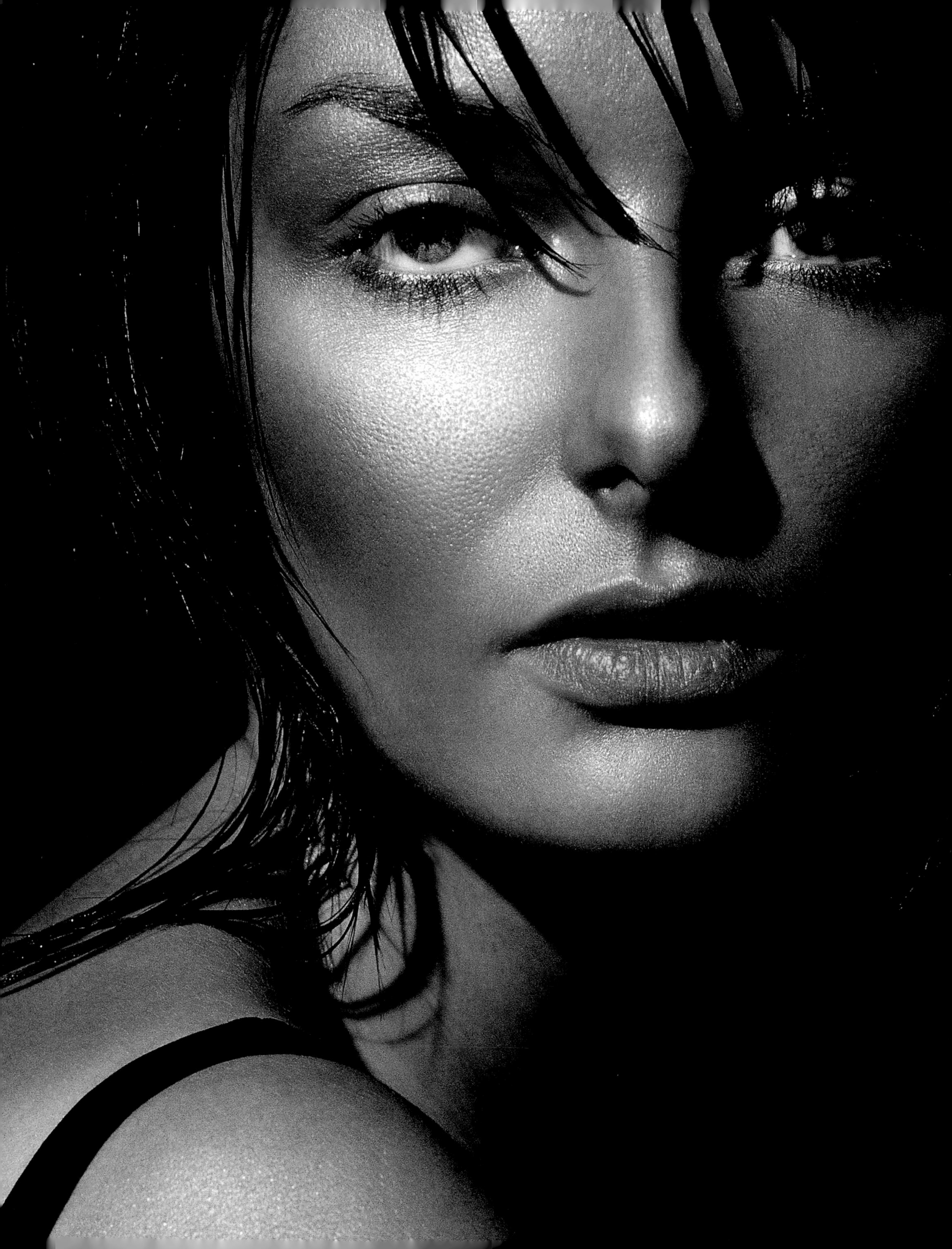

▶ **ADVICE FROM MARIE-THÉRÈSE LECCIA**
Professor of dermatology and photobiology at the University of Grenoble Hospital

The **signs of skin aging**—when skin sags or looks dull, when it begins to thicken, yellow, or become gaunt—are, for a surprising majority, linked to the sun. But you obviously must also account for environmental factors and lifestyle as well—a balanced diet and the least amount of toxins possible (alcohol, tobacco). The consequences of sunbathing are even worse if you smoke!

The key point of all these modifications is **oxidative stress,** the excessive production of the reactive elements of oxygen. These reactive molecules, which are derived from oxygen, are continually produced in our cells and under normal circumstances are eliminated. But when environmental variations (exposure to ultraviolet rays, temperature, toxins, and pollutants) occur, their production goes into overdrive and they become aggressive. They attack not only the cell itself (DNA, membranes, proteins) but also its surroundings—the entire tissue structure. Thus, at the dermis level, they damage the molecules that give good texture to skin, in particular, collagen and elastin fibers.

The overproduction of reactive molecules creates an imbalance in the defense mechanisms of skin (the antioxidant mechanisms that normally offer protection). This imbalance is what causes skin to age.

Hormone treatments during menopause can correct the hormonal changes that have an influence on skin (loss of tone, sagging) but also impact energy and well-being, potentially leading to a bout of depression, sleep disruption, or insomnia. They must be used carefully and under strict medical supervision.

The future of skin care

According to Professor Laurent Misery, the director of the skin neurobiology laboratory at the University of Brest, France, and specialist in the link between skin and the brain, the power of neurotransmitters offers exciting leads for the future of cosmetology.

Long live neuro-sensory research! You take care of yourself, use cosmetics, stay positive and happy, and focus on your well-being. This is great, but a massage all on its own is enough to release **dopamine**, the feel-good chemical in the brain. Without going into whether it works on your morale or on your stress, its results may be comparable to gentle drugs. If this is true, massage can offer a safe and healthy high since it triggers the very substances that work on the central nervous system.

THE PROMISES OF NEUROCOSMETICS

All the functions of skin are controlled by the nervous system and therefore connected to the mind. The **neurotransmitters** (chemical messengers) relay information between skin and the nervous system, and their role is to create a balance, except in certain dermatological illnesses or cosmetic skin inflammations, in which they actually activate skin problems (reactive skin).

Cosmetic formulations resulting from neuro-skin research acting on a neurotransmitter (either in one direction or the other) have the potential to teach us a great deal:

• **Anti-inflammatory** treatments can soothe sensitive skin and suppress itching and irritation.

• **Anti-hair-loss** treatments will stop the process of hair falling out.

• **Anti-cellulite** treatments can control the development of adipose cells via neurotransmitters, such as **VIP** (vasoactive intestinal peptide) and **leptin** (a protein given off by adult adipocytes), that report about reserves of adipose tissue to the brain. (A product resulting from the research on neuropeptides is already available on the market.)

• **Anti-age** spot treatments offer the ability to repigment the depigmented areas and vice versa. At the same time, however, it still remains impossible to reprogram the entire surface of skin to provide a completely new skin tone.

• **Anti-age** treatments can stimulate neurotransmitters that promote **the synthesis of collagen and elastin.**

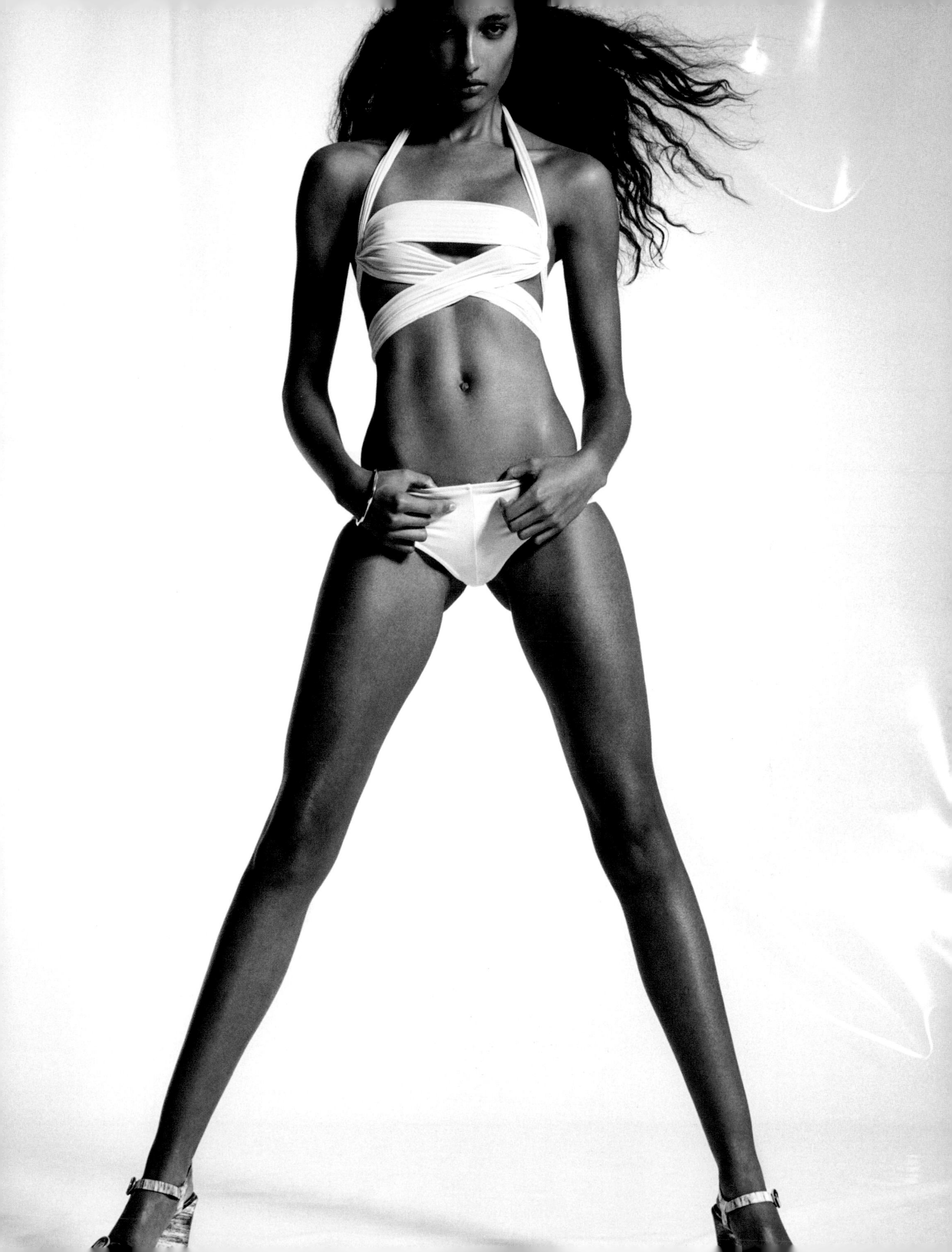

2 at the heart of your body

IMPORTANT POINTS

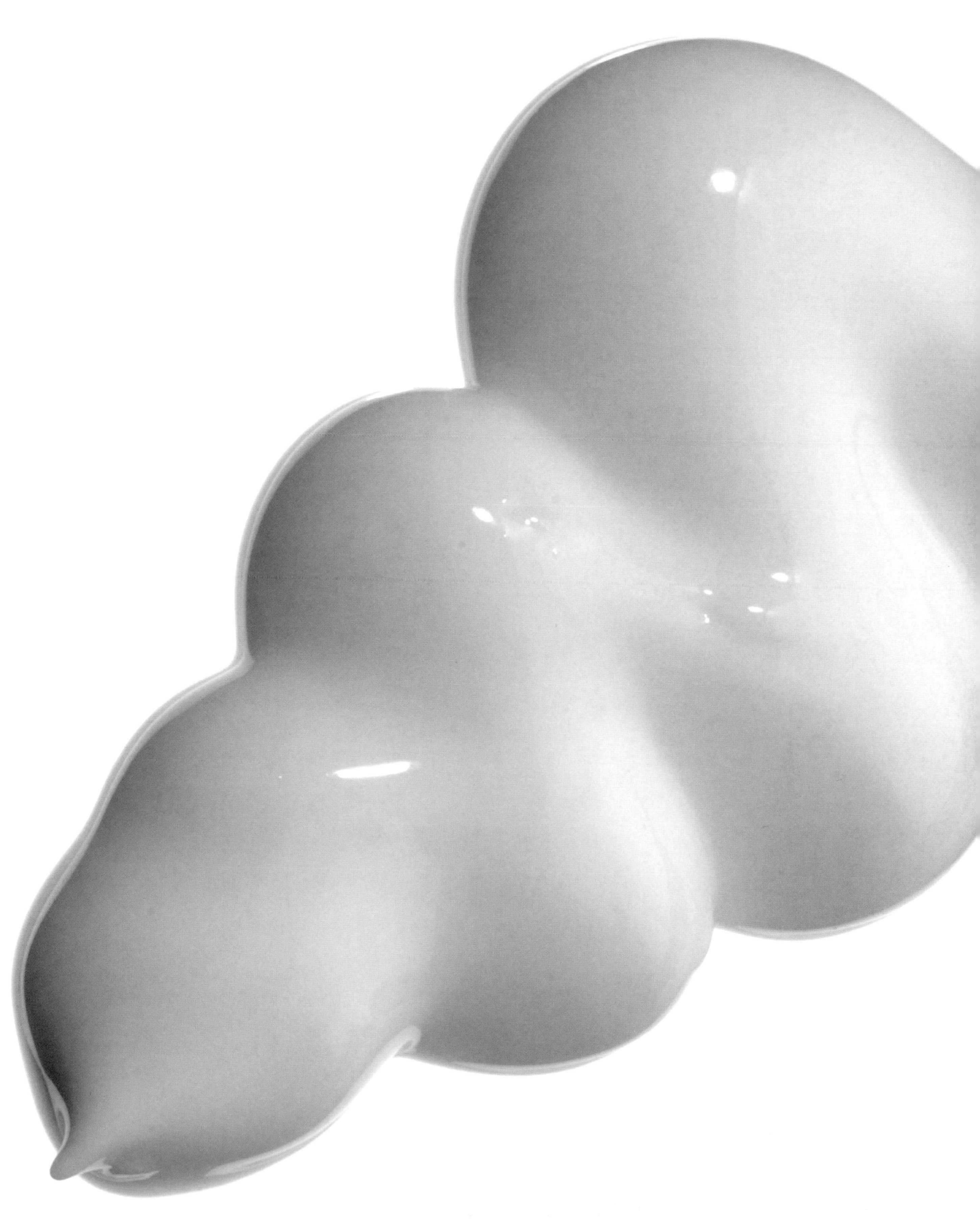

IMPORTANT POINTS

The reflection of your being is at the surface of your skin

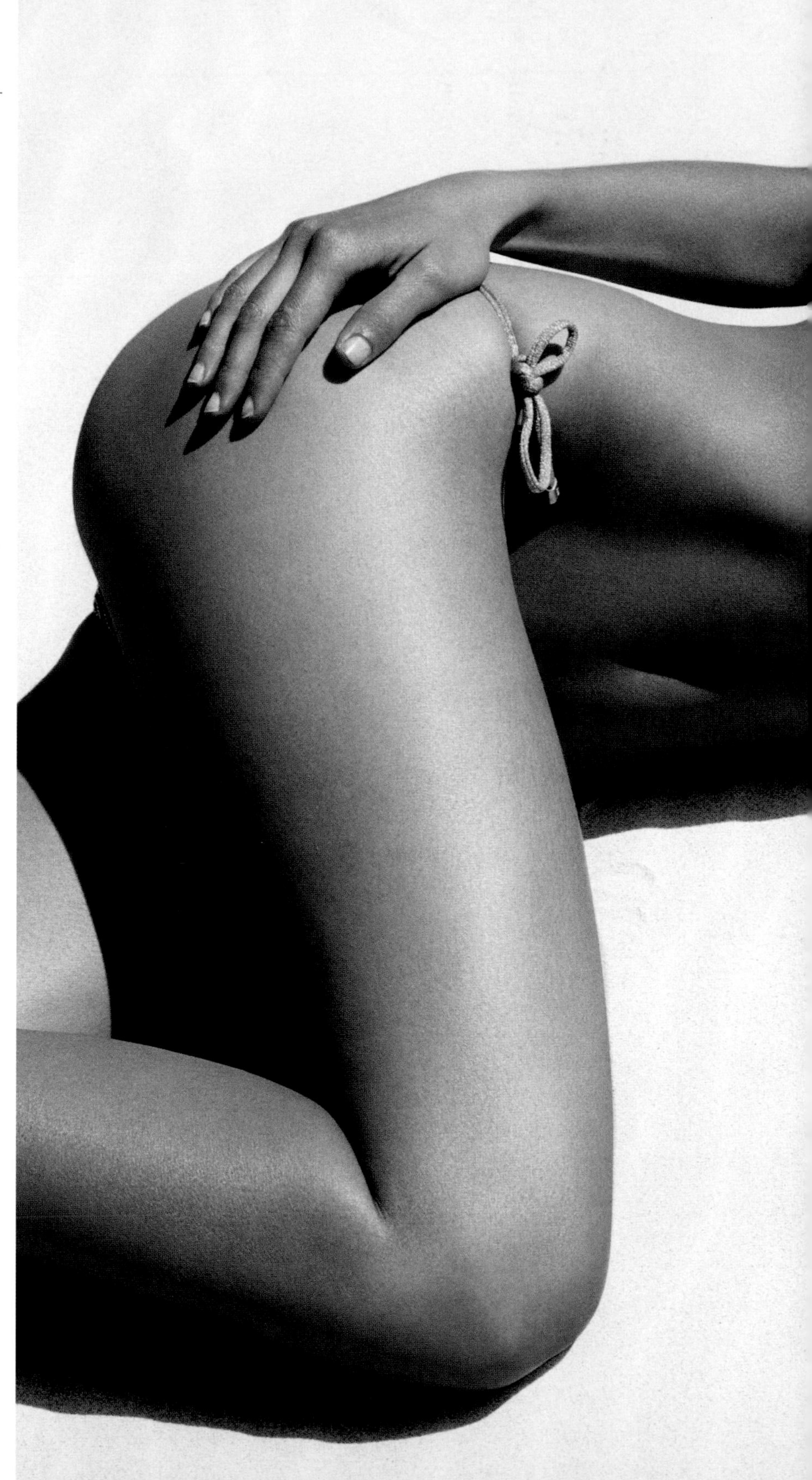

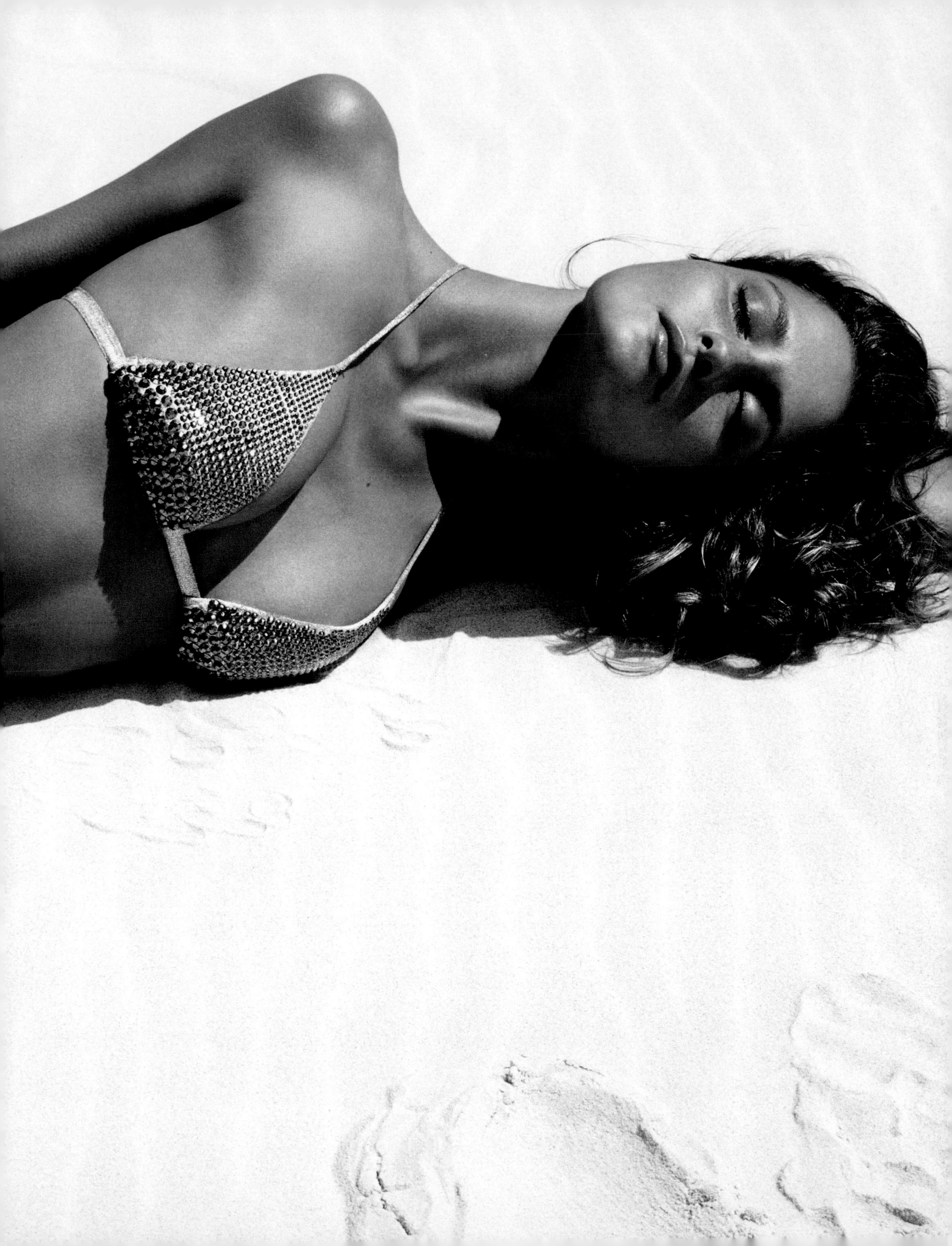

For graceful exposure... a pretty neck

Slender or strong, its line gives you the profile of a queen. It is also quite exposed and shows signs of age more than a smooth face is able to conceal!

A bare neck and nape will attract kisses. A dab of perfume there will attract even more.

ADVICE FROM A PERSONAL TRAINER

With your back straight, sitting in a chair, make 10 ovals in the air with the tip of your nose by moving your head from front to back, then rest for 10 seconds with your head tilted back. Then do this from right to left and then vertical to horizontal.

YOUNG NECK

Supple and graceful, with an incredible range of motion, it has the important task of holding your head up over the years . . . supporting no less than 11 pounds (the weight of your head) and protecting all its vital functions. This is an even more impressive challenge since its **muscle structure is less dense than that of the face and its skin is as thin as that on the eyelids** and contains very little sebum. To prevent muscular degeneration, you must not neglect your neck in your **daily care routine** of hydrating and nourishing. Even if it doesn't wrinkle, it can lose its elasticity and take on a saggy look. Therefore, every morning and night, use ultranourishing skin care products enriched with astringent agents that will tighten skin and envelop it in a protective film.

Double chin SOS treatments to thin and drain will help to reshape the oval, while lifting and refirming treatments reinforce the tissue underneath. **Skin-tightening** treatments can improve the consistency of the skin's structure and revitalize it.

ROYAL BEARING

Stand up straight with your elbows in your palms, behind your head, and shoulder blades tight; imagine you are a sovereign ready to put the crown on your head. And don't forget the gym (see page 167)!

HAIR FOR ALL NECK TYPES

A long neck looks best with a medium-length cut and pretty necklaces. A **short** neck needs a bare nape, but avoid round-necked shirts. For a **thick** neck, wear your hair up and make the most of tops with deep V-necks and dangling earrings.

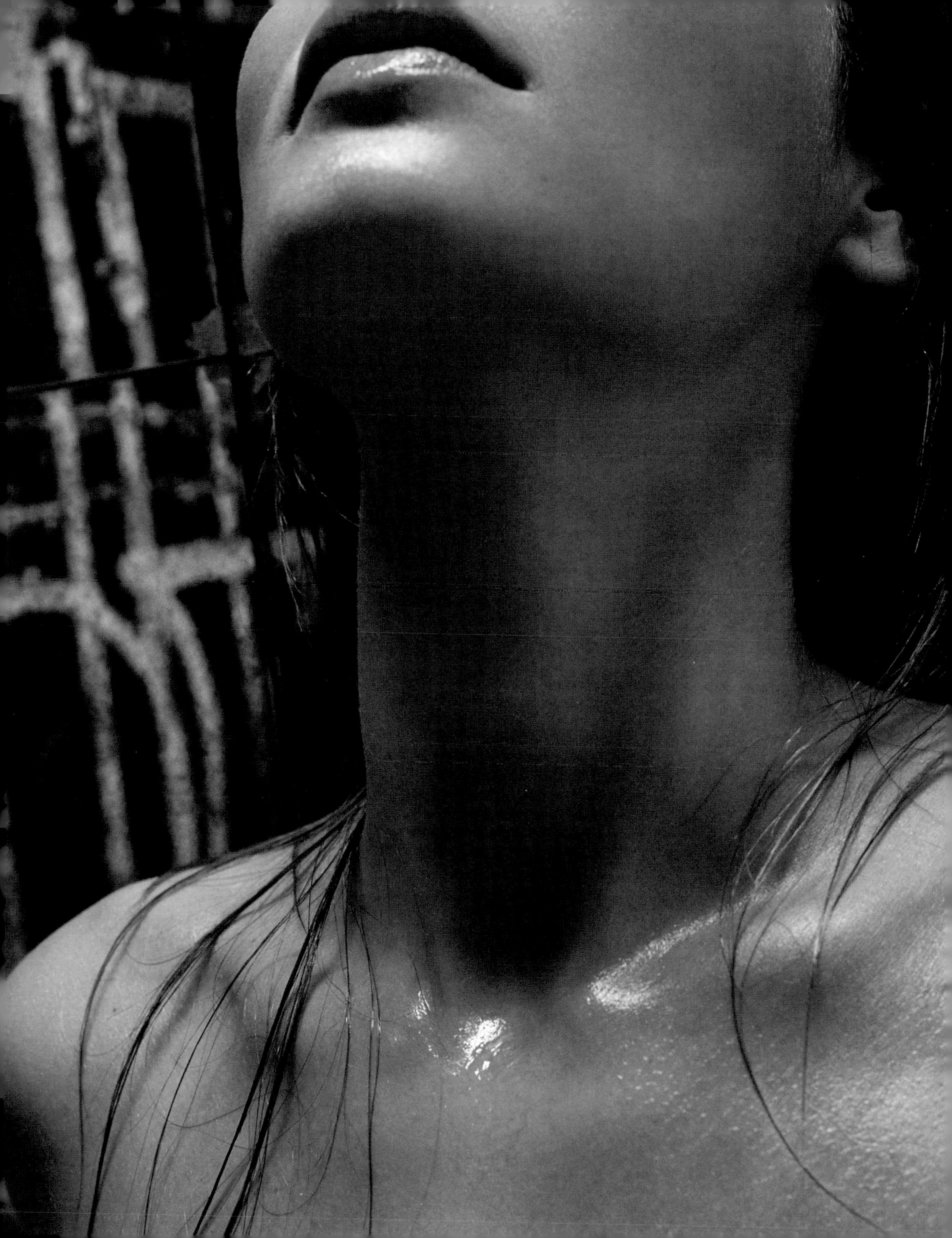

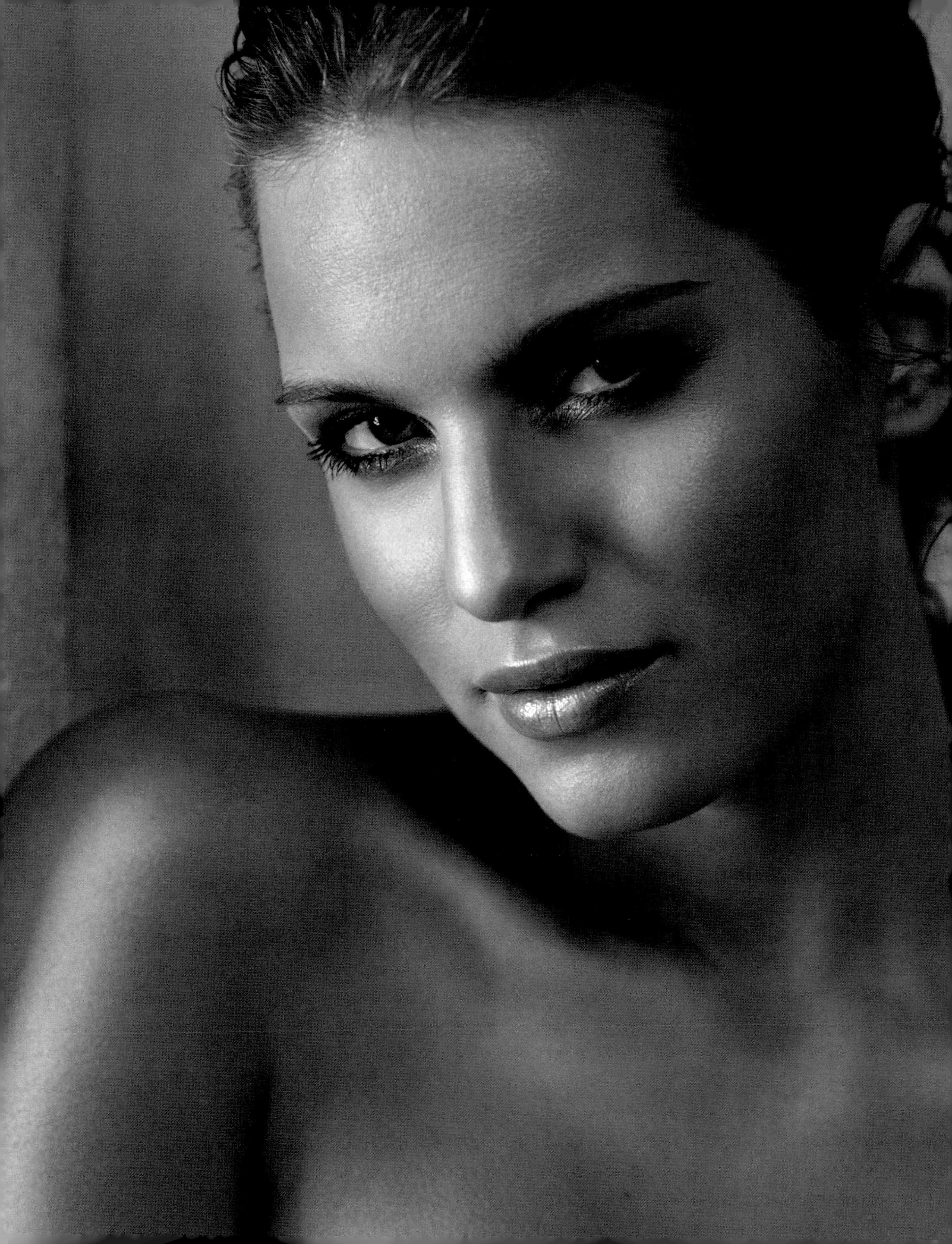

Perfect shoulders

They emphasize the shape of your silhouette, uphold the entire framework of your body, define your movement, and shape your posture. One single motto: Shoulders back!

The Trend is for Squared, Sculpted Shoulders

You're smart to hold your head high on your shoulders. It's difficult to imagine a more ingenious plan than this structure, with its incredible complexity, connecting the shoulder blades and the humerus and kept supple by a group of ligaments.

Beautiful shoulders, solid and well developed, frame the silhouette and help to keep it tall.

Good posture—shoulders back and relaxed—opens the thorax and makes breathing easier. To keep them nice and straight, stretch and gently roll your shoulders.

There are many exercises to tone shoulders and make them more limber. In sports, everything depends on their form.

If your shoulders are too narrow, swimming is the best sport for you to strengthen them; but tennis is great as well.

If your shoulders are too broad, work on your dancer legs or practice skating, skiing, or rollerblading.

Shoulders Tall

Square shoulders Tank tops, bustiers, boatnecks, and plunging necklines will make you look like a movie star and showcase your shoulders.

Sloping shoulders With some help from shoulder pads, which give a bit of volume, you can cheat and give the impression of square shoulders.

At the computer, move the mouse while keeping your forearms flat on the desk. Otherwise, you will cause approximately 11 pounds of tension on the muscles, which will eventually result in neck pain.

ADVICE FROM A PERSONAL TRAINER

SELF-MASSAGES

- **Starting at the neck, knead the upper part of your shoulder between your palm and fingers, focusing on the tighter areas, all the way down your arms.**
- **Massage your shoulder blades with the tips of your fingers in little circles.**

TENDONITIS, one of the most common forms of pain in the shoulders, is due to an inflammation of the tendons that surround the joints.

Décolletage revealed

Suggestive or suggested, plunging or push-up, décolletage is the focus of fashion and is becoming more and more prominent in every season.

Circular massage using the tips of your fingers, from the base of your breasts all the way to your chin, will improve circulation and tone the skin tissue. Exfoliate to bring a healthy glow back to your décolletage. Skin care treatments with a base of fruit acids work very nicely.

FRAGILE—HANDLE WITH CARE!

This area is very sensitive to UV rays, and the décolletage is one of the sun's favorite points of attack. Without enough protection, too much sun exposure creates visible damage to the elastin and collagen in the form of vertical striations.

SHAPE UP!

We can't develop muscle tone in our breasts because there are none there! However, we can strengthen the pectoral muscles, which form the base for our chest and open up the thoracic cavity, to make our breasts look better.

Getting a better view

- For red carpet–ready décolletage in the summer, use oils and glitter.
- To create the impression of volume, dust a bit of bronzing powder between your breasts.
- For extra cleavage, slip small, invisible silicon inserts into your bra.
- To flatter a small chest, wear V-necks and necklaces.

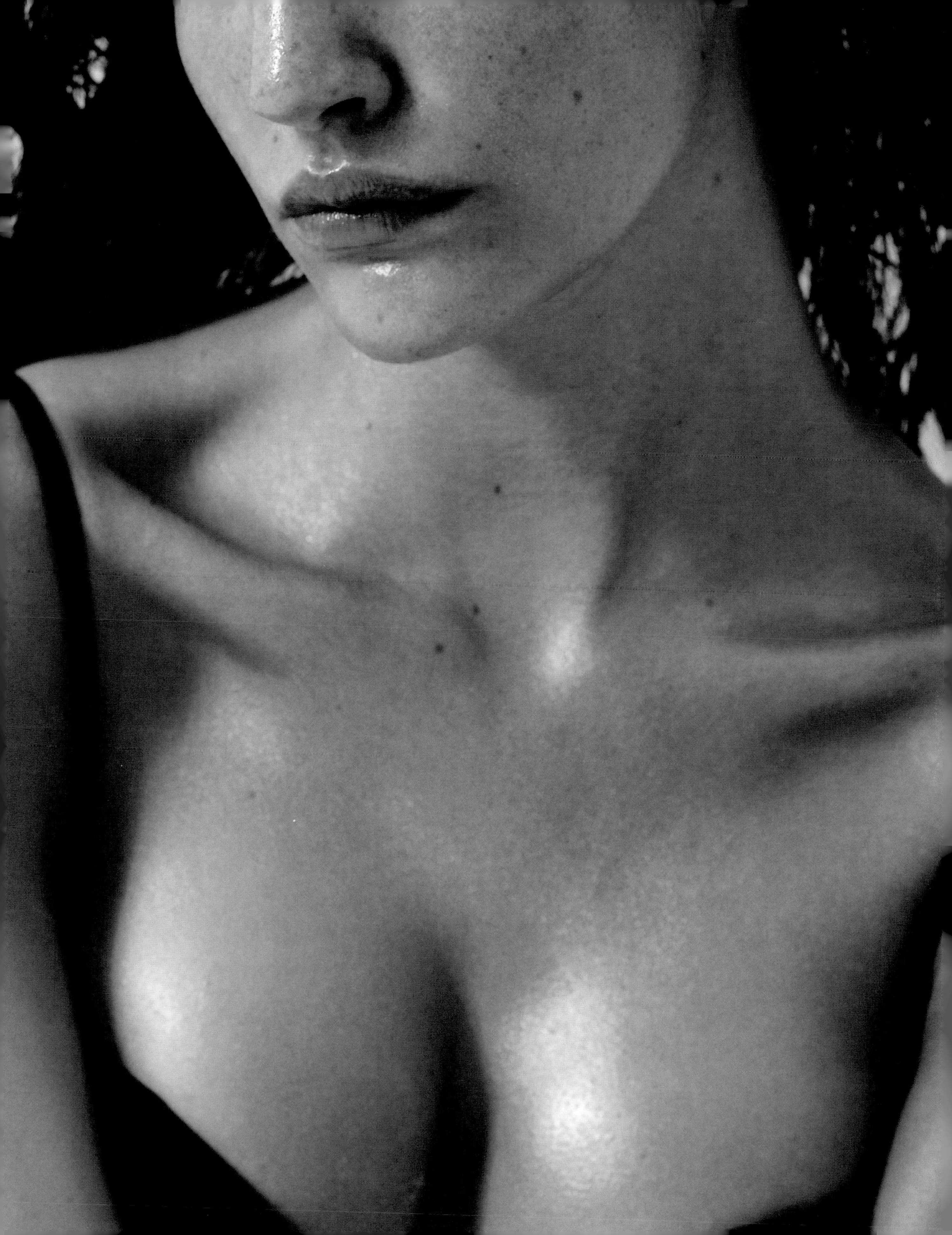

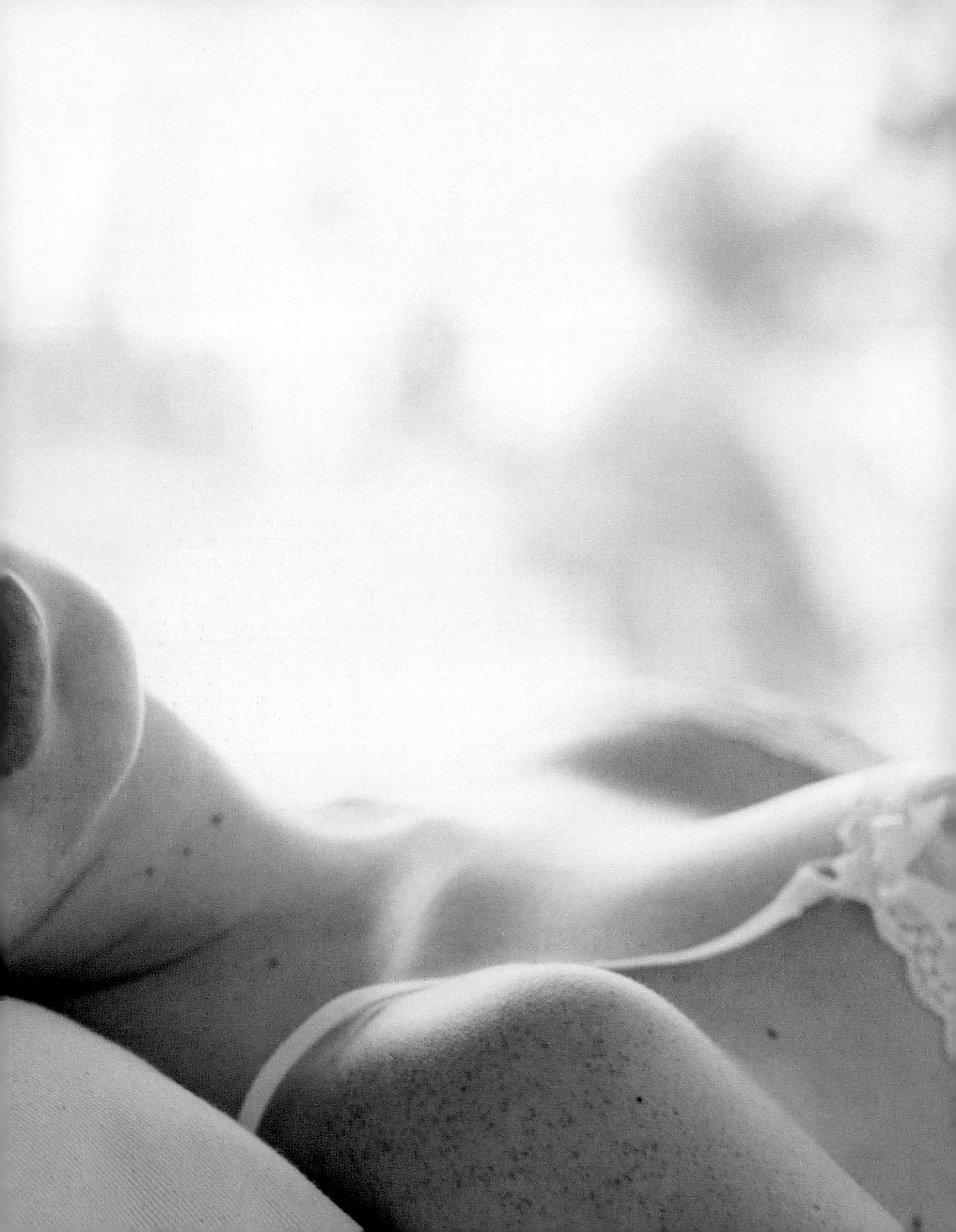

Your breasts: the height of seduction

Apple- or pear-shaped, forbidden fruits or reclaimed symbols of femininity, from the smallest to the fullest, they have never before been flaunted so proudly!

SKIN: NATURE'S BRA

Your breasts contain no muscle and are simply "parked" on your thorax: only the envelope of skin that surrounds the mammary gland helps to counteract their weight. That's why it's so important to pay some attention to that skin!

FRESH WATER EVERY DAY!

Shower treatments are indispensable: everyday, splash your breasts with warm, then cool, then cold water while gently massaging them. This encourages circulation and stimulates breast tissue. Excessive heat is their biggest enemy!

Hydrate and tone this fragile area daily using **circular massage.** Refirming treatments and boosting masks will help stimulate the production of collagen and elastin.

GOOD POSITION

Sit straight when seated, with your shoulders pulled back behind you, to help prevent your breasts from sagging.

SUPPORT GROUP

Everyday bra A full-coverage bra will keep even a large chest in place and prevent bouncing when you walk.

Sports bra A good sports bra should have reinforced and padded shoulder straps.

Special occasion bra Specialty bras provide beautiful curves and cleavage.

KEY POINTS

The **back** of your bra must not ride up; the **cups** must be adjusted perfectly, neither digging in or cutting off circulation nor making creases when you lift your arms. Underwires are great as long as they do not pinch or hurt. The **straps,** placed on the top of the shoulder, must not leave indentations or red marks on the skin.

ADVICE FROM A PERSONAL TRAINER

Sports that build up back muscles and the pectorals (swimming, handball) are good for your breasts, as are the following target exercises:

- **Sitting up straight with a two-pound weight in each hand, knees folded in to chest, without arching your back, bring your arms down slowly behind your head while exhaling, then bring them back up slowly (repeat 20 times).**
- **Flat on your stomach, arms slightly outstretched, palms of your hands on the floor, and toes pointed, raise your entire body parallel to the floor.**
- **On your knees, arms in front of you with your hands on the floor, bring your torso down to the floor and push it back up slowly.**

Beautiful back

You can also attract attention from behind using the body part that carries all your stress and fatigue. Muscular, relaxed, and massaged, our back begs us not to forget about it.

THE VERTEBRAL COLUMN: OUR SUPPORT BEAM

The **joints** adapt to all ranges of motion: stretching, twisting, and all the rhythms of breathing. The entire spinal column is held together by ligaments and groups of muscles that package together this mechanical and aesthetic marvel.

Seducing with your back, displaying your streamlined muscles, is a sign of power.

THE SKIN ON YOUR BACK

Even though it's thicker than the skin on your face, it also needs purification and hydration. Exfoliation and massage are important, even if it's just smoothing on hydrating cream, making sure not to miss an inch. A brush with a long handle and soft bristles will help you exfoliate and gently massage your back in the shower.

VISIT TO THE SPA

Purifying and cleansing treatments (with steam, for example), to keep pimples and blackheads in check, and masks (clay, mud, or seaweed) for deep cleaning, should be performed before hydrating. A massage will help to promote circulation.

EXERCISES FOR A BEAUTIFUL BACK

The **backstroke** (which elongates the muscle), **front stroke** (to maintain the muscle), and **volleyball** and **basketball** (for stretching, which enhances the silhouette) are all excellent for your back. **Yoga** and **gyrotonic** exercises harmoniously develop muscles, all while relaxing your body and reducing tension and stress.

- Sleep on your back or on your side with a small pillow supporting your neck to keep the vertebral column aligned.
- At work, arrange your space so that the computer screen is at eye level and regularly stretch your shoulders back.
- In the car, keep your back comfortably supported, knees level with your hips, and two hands on the steering wheel with the arms parallel.

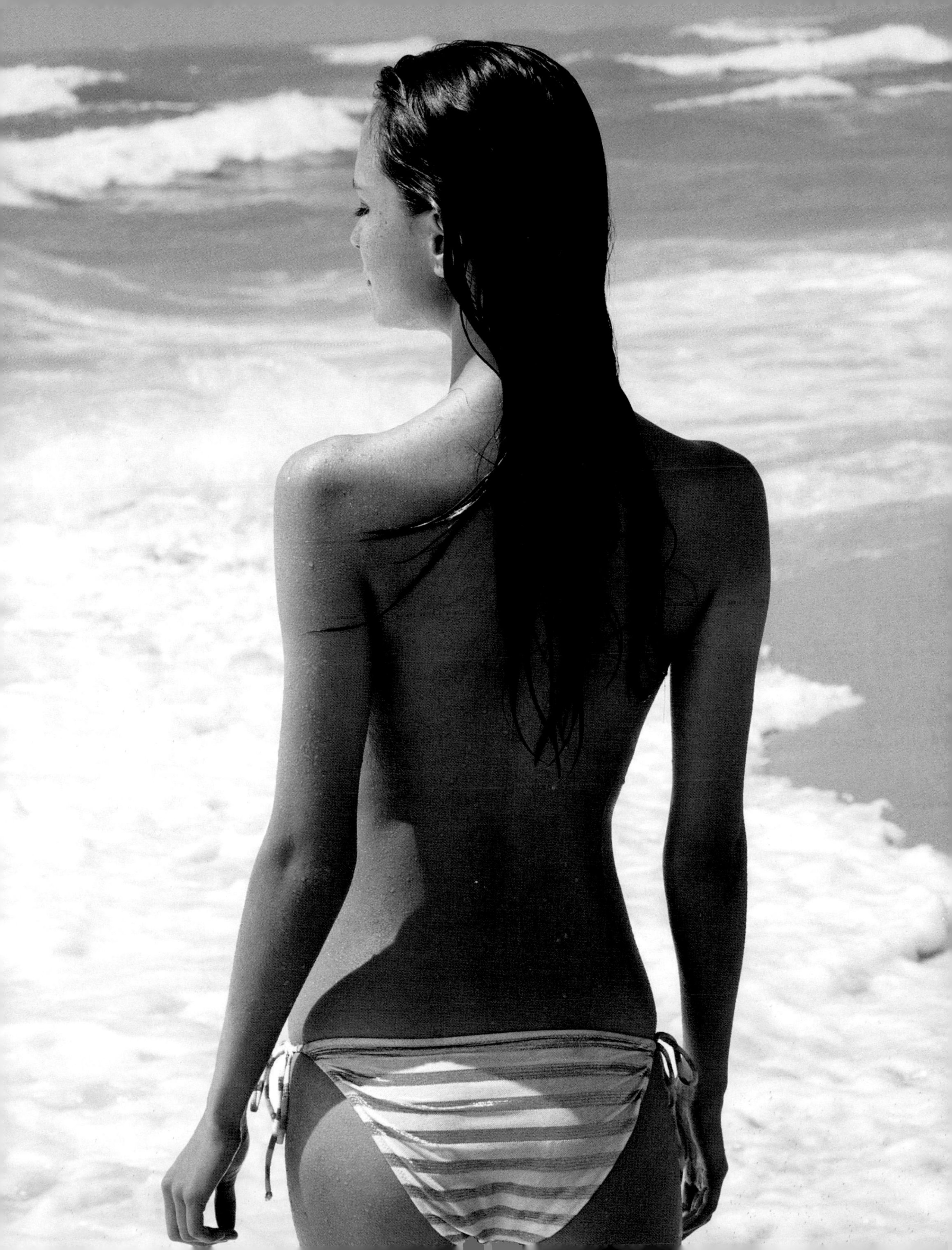

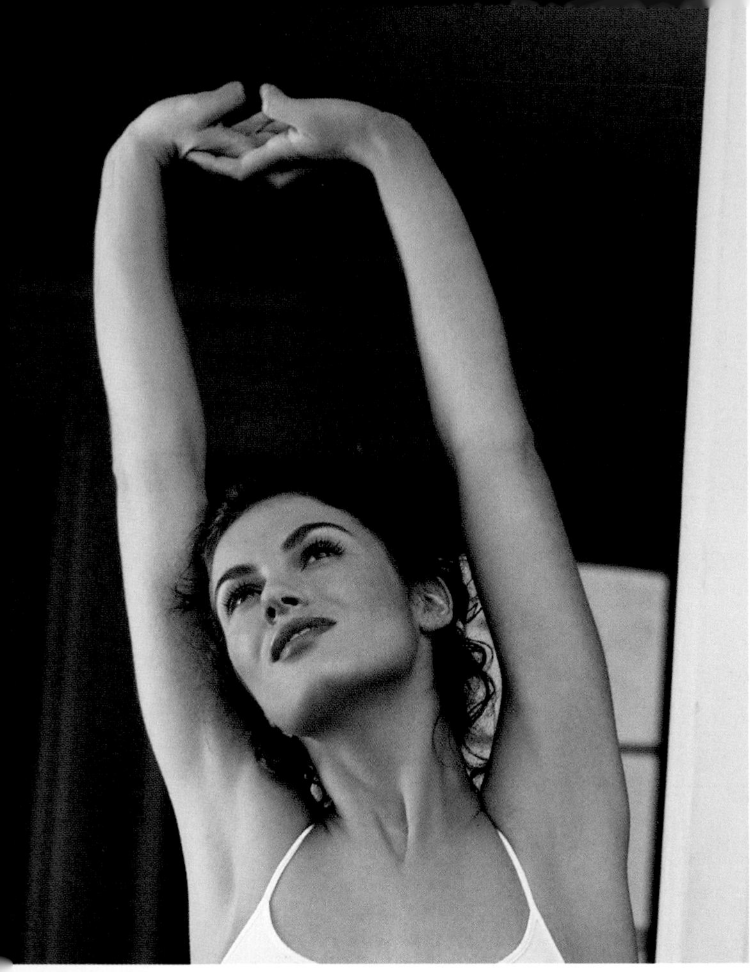

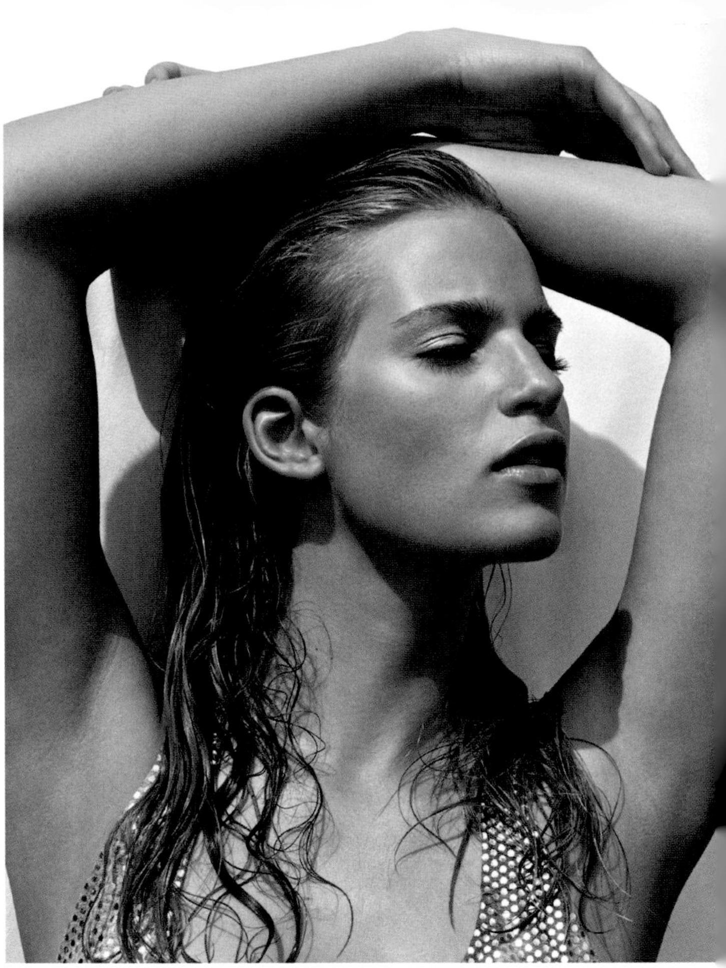

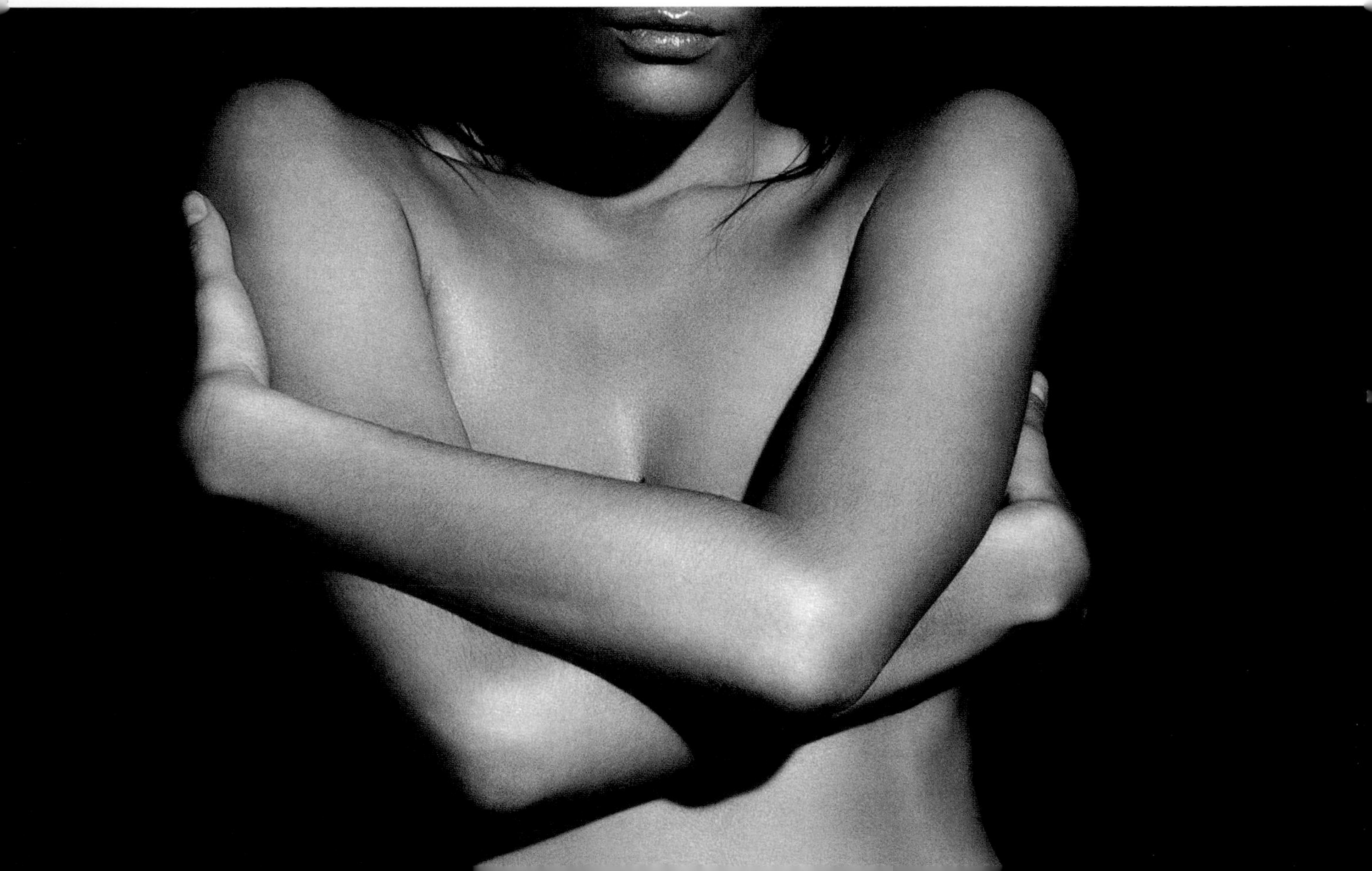

Embrace your arms

You can't always hide your arms or keep them crossed. Although the incredible arms of an Olympic swimmer may be an impossible dream, you can still have pretty arms that will give you a great silhouette.

PRETTY, FEMININE ARMS

Bare arms are seen at every occasion—even more reason to keep them looking great. Body language is essential to the image that you project, and the language of your arms speaks volumes.

The **ultrathin skin,** especially on the back of your arms, requires extra attentive care that nourishes, firms (this is one of the first places to show signs of sagging), improves the density, and protects. **Exfoliate** the back of your arm with a textured glove or cloth (bristles are too harsh), then massage the area thoroughly after showering, moving from wrist to elbow and then elbow to shoulder. **Cellulite** can be curbed in this area by using **rolling** and **circular massage** along with anticellulite treatments.

Elbows love hydrating and nourishing creams. There is nothing worse than wrinkly and rough elbows, the result of friction with clothing and cold weather, which promotes dryness.

Downy hairs on your arms can be pretty, especially when they turn golden in the summer, unless you have too much. Bleaching is preferable to removing dark hair.

EXERCISES FOR GREAT ARMS

Your arms respond much more quickly than your thighs to getting in shape. Sculpt your arms in one month? It's no joke! These exercises firm the underlying tissues and shape up flabby arms. Fatty tissue in your arms melts away much more quickly than it does in your legs. The exercises in the column to the right require a pair of adjustable-weight dumbbells.

Dancing will help to sculpt your figure and promote graceful movement. **Tennis**, **swimming**, and **yoga** are also great for your arms.

ADVICE FROM A PERSONAL TRAINER

FOR THINNER ARMS, use six-pound weights in each hand (any heavier and you will bulk up):

- Seated on a chair, with your knees bent, legs slightly apart, arms loose and fully extended the length of your body, slowly bring your outstretched arm up to the height of your shoulder and bring it down again slowly (do two sets of 20 for each arm).

FOR ARMS OF STEEL, use three-pound weights in each hand to tone your triceps:

- Seated with your back comfortably supported in a chair, raise your outstretched left arm level to your ear.
- Bend your elbow, bringing your forearm toward the nape of your neck, then out straight again.
- Repeat this for the right side (do three sets of 30).

Healthy hands and fingers

They communicate more through body language than through their beauty. The most extraordinary tool that nature has put at our disposal deserves all of our attention.

Show of hands! A study published by the American Society of Plastic Surgeons (ASPS) in June 2006 revealed that the best way to guess someone's age is to look at the hands. The good news is, using nail polish and wearing jewelry make them look younger! **Your nails** grow a little over a tenth of an inch every month (they renew themselves completely every four to six months), but their growth speeds up in the summer months. If you are right-handed, the nails on that hand will grow faster.

DAILY MAINTENANCE REQUIRED!

Your hands are matrices of superb complexity composed of the flexible joint of the wrist, five metacarpal bones, the fingers (with two phalanges for the thumb and three for the others), and their many small muscles that give them strength and precision. The abductor muscles allow you to spread your fingers, and the adductor muscles bring them back together.

The **thick skin on the palm,** which has no sebaceous glands, and the **thin skin on the back of the hand** result in a thirst and a dryness that is aggravated even more by frequent hand washing. Keep your hands beautiful with frequent gentle exfoliation and daily massage using **special hydrating creams** that nourish and prevent wrinkles **(as well as hangnails).** UV protection is required every day, since the sun's rays cause premature aging.

Special night repair Use a gentle hand mask, applied in a thick layer, and then put on a pair of cotton gloves.

Nail care Your nails and the half moon at the base require constant care. Use a strengthening base coat and a protective polish.

SOS for brittle nails Place your nails in a bowl of warm almond oil for 10 minutes.

Cold hands To encourage circulation, raise your hands in the air and massage from the tips of your fingers down to your wrists.

YOUTHFUL HANDS

Plastic surgery, lasers, and chemical peels can all erase age spots, while injectible fillers can bring back some baby-soft plumpness.

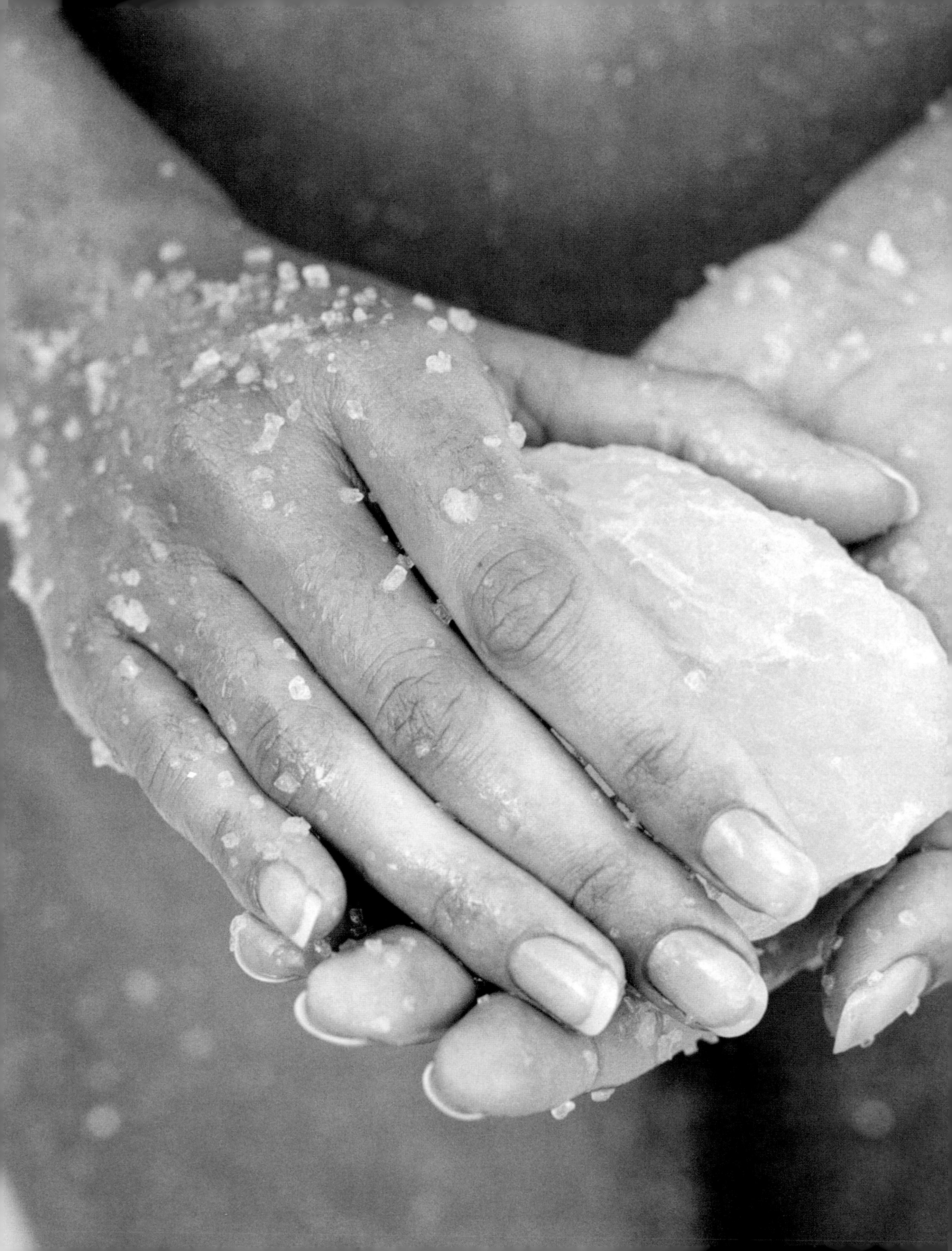

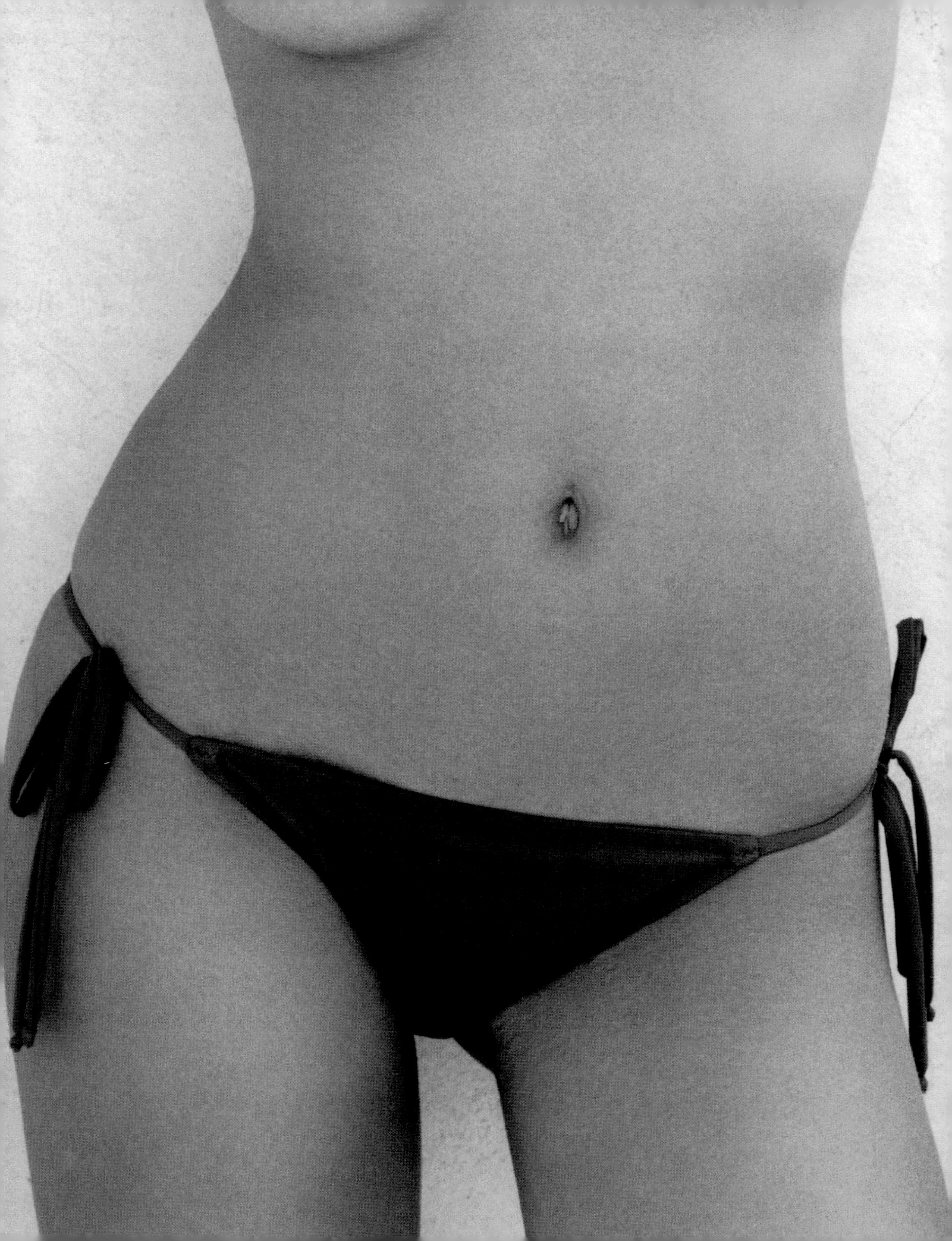

Abdomen: the issue of your waist

Flat abs or a cute little tummy, your waist leads the rest of your body in the dance of seduction. And fashion trends featuring low waistlines bring it out in the open.

Wasp Waist Your waist thins out at puberty and thickens at menopause. Situated about 1.5 inches above our navel, this magic line cinches in our figure. The waist has always been a symbol of femininity, but its size depends greatly on heredity. Unfortunately, you may be predisposed to a thicker waist—or thighs!

NO REST FOR THE ABS!

The female anatomy is predisposed to extra padding around the middle: this is the promised land for adipocytes. To succeed in our quest for a flat stomach, we must focus on two groups of four muscle groups (the rectus abdominis, the internal and external obliques, and the transverse) that make up the famous six pack. These muscle groups support the abdomen and protect our organs, all while shoring up the lower back and helping the spinal column do its job. Aside from detox cures made of green tea and special diets, working your abs daily is the only way to shape them into the enviable six pack, by reducing fatty tissue and sculpting the muscles. And you can still get great abs even after having a baby, once the perineum is healed.

Target your abs (and vary your routine so you don't get bored) and massage them with a **formula that drains the fluids** (one that contains caffeine, bitter orange, and calcium), lifting the skin and sculpting your midsection.

Massage rules! At home or in the spa, you can conquer cellulite at your waistline by repetitive massage, trapping it and rolling it between your fingers, alternating between waves and concentric circles.

Eat slowly, drink green tea, breathe deeply: this is the winning combination for toning your abs.

ADVICE FROM A PERSONAL TRAINER

CONSIDER YOUR ABS WHEN YOU'RE OUT AND ABOUT

As you're walking around, imagine you are sucking in your navel, reducing your sides, and tightening your buttocks!

THE KING OF THE ABS:

- On your back, with your legs up vertically, breathe in deeply and then raise your chest as you exhale, looking at the ceiling so that you lift your back without rolling your neck. At the end of the exhale, return to the floor, bringing your head and navel back into alignment.

SECRET FOR FLAT ABS:

- Rowing and swimming the backstroke to boost abdominal blood flow
- Pilates and yoga
- Salsa—the best dance for flat abs!

Bottoms up: your best behind

Do not underestimate your assets; beautiful backsides have changed the face of the world!

EVERYONE'S FAVORITE: A BOMBSHELL BOTTOM!

We love round, high, curvy bottoms that seem to never sag or droop. Good news—**it's the quality of skin, the true natural covering** of your behind, that gives this perky profile. The most important thing to remember for this area is to stimulate the circulation and skin tone, which is much easier than changing nature.

ARCH YOUR BACK

Small, medium, and large gluteus muscles A trio of muscles form the curves of your dreams: the small and the medium (abductor) gluteus muscles are on the sides, shaping the hips, and the large gluteus muscle shapes your buttocks. To learn where these are found, here are three body types:

Large behind (endomorphic) A spectacular small of the back that's quickly contrasted by the added weight of buttocks carrying too much fatty tissue results in a pear-shaped behind.

Flat behind (mesomorphic) This is firm and well sculpted, but not quite full.

Underdeveloped (ectomorphic) You will need to find your curves through targeted exercises.

THE BOTTOM LINE IN CARE

Rolling massage combined with firming and fluid-draining treatments work wonderfully. Daily massage, always from bottom to top, will help lift your profile.

ADVICE FROM A PERSONAL TRAINER

TRAINING PLAN

- Tighten the muscles in your bottom frequently throughout the day, each time holding the contraction longer and longer.
- When you walk, take large steps, pushing off with the back leg.
- Boycott elevators and escalators.

LIFT IT UP

- Stretched out on your right side, with your right leg bent, torso leaning in toward the floor and supported by your hands, extend your left leg with your toes pointing down. Breathe in deeply, and when you exhale, stretch your left leg behind you without arching your back (repeat 25 times on each leg).
- On your back, slowly raise your legs vertically, toes pointing upward (repeat 25 times).

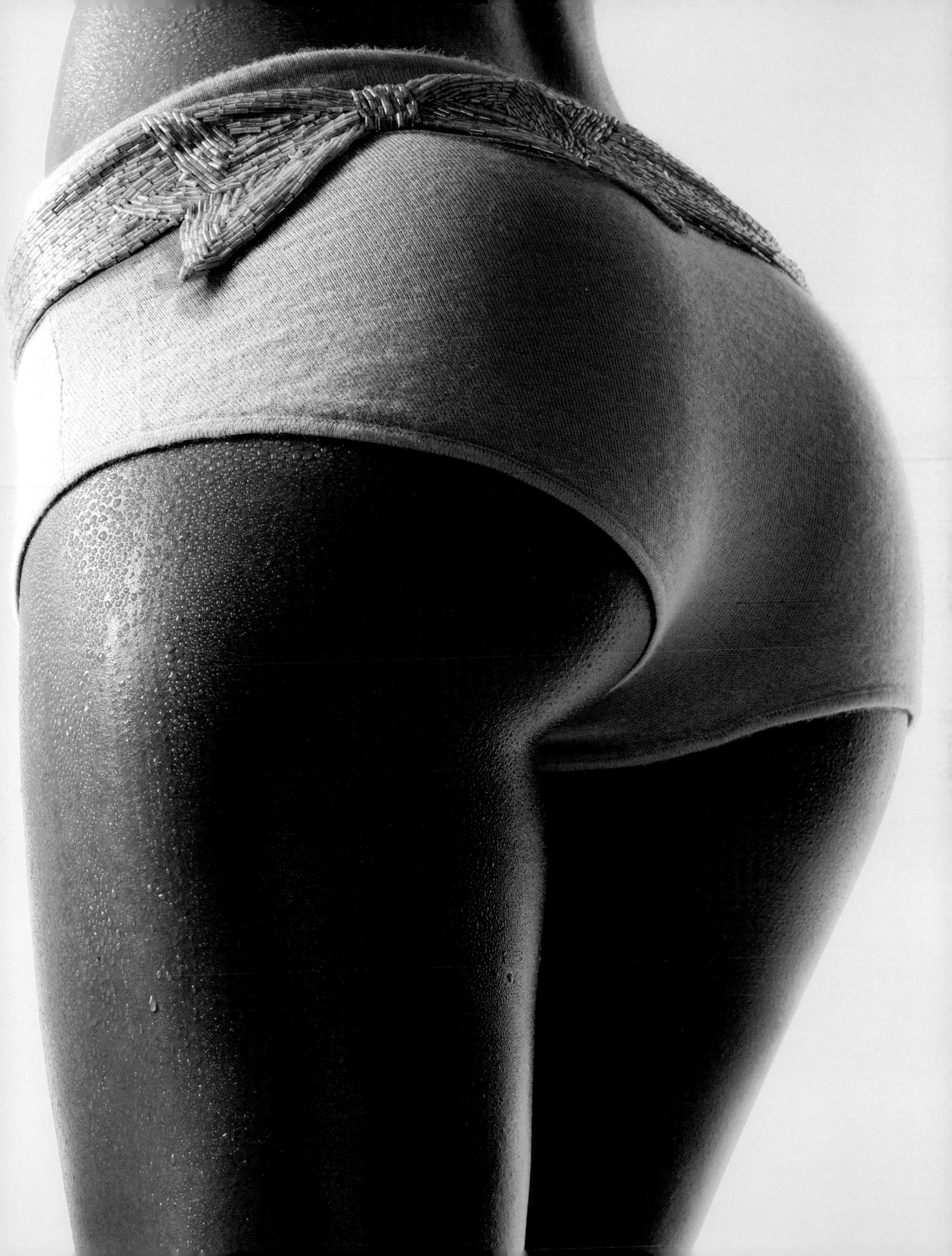

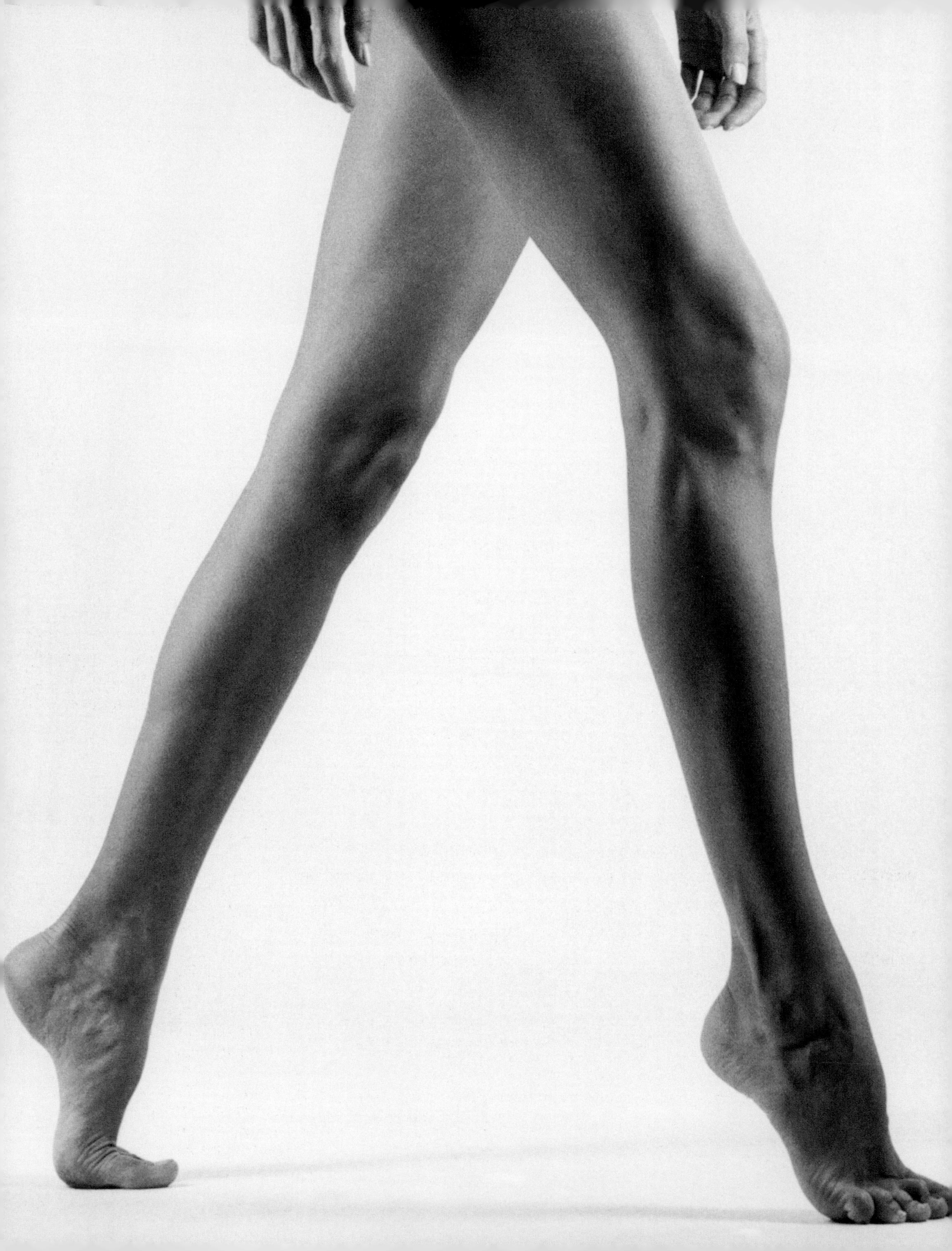

Legs of your dreams

Pillars of femininity, columns of a temple...
The superlatives accorded to our legs set the bar very high—
even higher as skirts get shorter.

PERFECT LEGS

Architecturally, our legs move our body. The **thigh,** attached to the torso at the hip by the neck of the femur, features a network of incredibly powerful muscles (quadriceps, adductors, and hamstrings in the back). It extends to the **knee,** which forms the joint that connects to the **calf** (via the tibia and the fibula), which then extends to the ankle. This amazing combination of bone and muscle has created champions.

TAPERING THIGHS, SHAPELY CALVES, SLENDER ANKLES

Forty-four inch long perfect legs are unfortunately out of reach if you were not born with them. The dream of willowy thighs, flawless calves, and tiny ankles lures us like the prospect of a miracle. Thankfully, there are resources to help nature along:

• Plants that help **drain fluid** or work as protective agents (ginkgo biloba; red wine grapes; cypress; melilot, also known as sweet clover; dandelion).

• **Anticellulite formulas**, which are becoming more effective and easier to apply. You can also benefit from massage, working from the soles of the feet to the ankles, the back of the calves, and the thighs all the way to the hips and buttocks, using circular strokes.

• Sports, such as **walking, biking,** and **ballet bar exercises.**

GOOD NEWS

• Compression stockings are available in graduated versions.

• Very flattering self-tanning lotions (that hydrate and slim at the same time) are available year-round.

• If you have the instep for it, you add nearly four inches to your calf by wearing heels of that height (be sure to use the nightly massage found on page 180!).

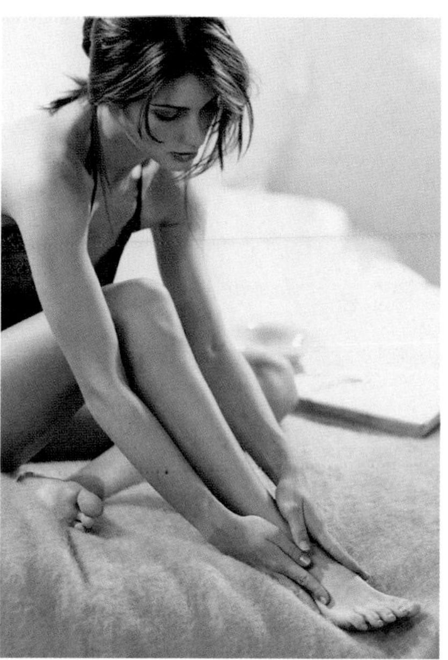

The enemies of your legs:

• Being sedentary
• Long periods of standing
• Excess weight
• Too much heat (avoid hot baths!)
• Clothes that are too tight

ADVICE FROM A PERSONAL TRAINER

FOR BEAUTIFUL THIGHS

Standing upright, knees straight, feet apart, pull in your stomach, tighten your buttocks, and extend your left leg, toes pointed, out in front of you. Hold this pose for two seconds and bring your leg back down to the floor (repeat 25 times on each leg).

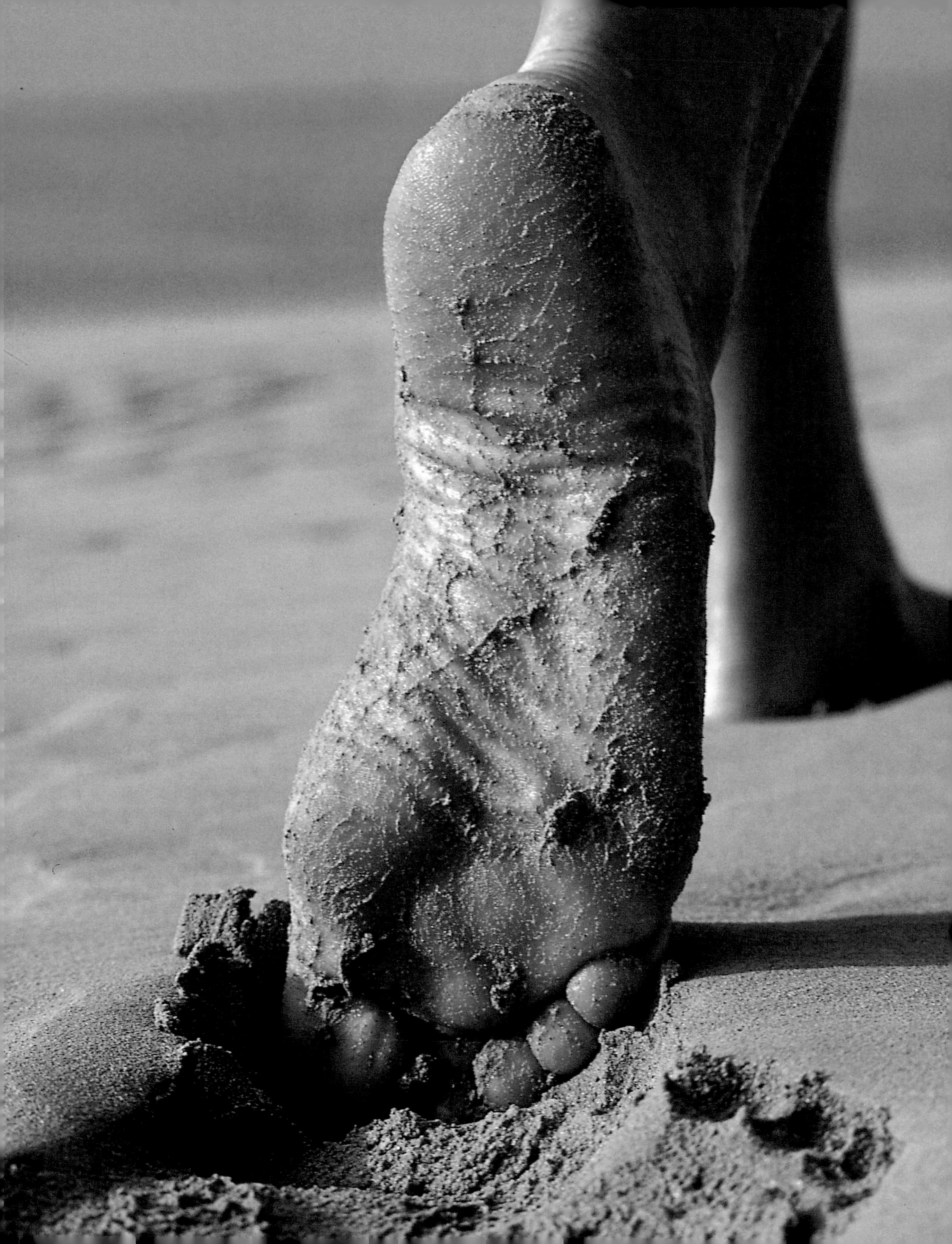

The world at your feet

They constantly support and transport us. Advice from podiatrist Ari Darmon keeps them beautiful.

Our feet bravely carry the weight of our body (multiplied by two when we run!) on their **26 bones** connected by a brilliant complex of muscles and tendons that ensure stability; a subcutaneous shock absorber of fatty tissue separates them from the ground. When the foot is irritated, **hyperkeratosis** plays a protective role in the form of a corn or a callous. The **sole of the foot** and the palm of the hand are the only two hairless areas of skin on the body, but, unfortunately, they are not also free of perspiration!

FLAT FOOT OR ARCHED FOOT?

The length of your foot corresponds to the height of your arch. For example, if your foot is 10 inches long, then your arch should be approximately 1 inch off the ground. If it's higher off the ground, your foot is arched. If it's lower, your foot is flat—the case for 80 percent of us. The opposable thumb that has become the big toe directs our walking.

The Toenails, which, just like the nails on your hands, are part of the **superficial** body growth system, need to be nourished. Blood travels the farthest to reach them, so the toes are the last served. When **circulation** is poor, especially in the legs, the toenails suffer, become striated, and break.

Shoes help keep your feet in balance, so it is important to choose them wisely based on the shape of your foot and how you will be using them. Blend aesthetics and function. **It's not normal for your feet to hurt!**

Shape! Egyptian (with a long big toe), **Roman** (squared, with the first three toes the same length), or **Greek** (the second toe is the longest), the **shape of the foot** must be considered when you buy shoes, otherwise you'll wind up with corns, calluses, bunions, and other foot problems. The only solution is a visit to the podiatrist!

Once a week (but not more, since rubbing stimulates corns),
• file with a pumice stone and then use a gentle exfoliant.

Every day, after the shower or bath to hydrate, you need to use lotion or cream. Using cream daily will keep the skin on your foot as supple as possible.

Pedicure must-haves:
• Nail clippers (but don't clip too far down on the sides) and nail scissors
• Tweezers
• Orange stick for nails and cuticles
• Nail buffer
• Hydrating cream

ADVICE FROM A PODIATRIST

Walk barefooted on the sand: this is one of the best exercises for massaging the soles of the feet and allows all the joints in your feet to move freely.

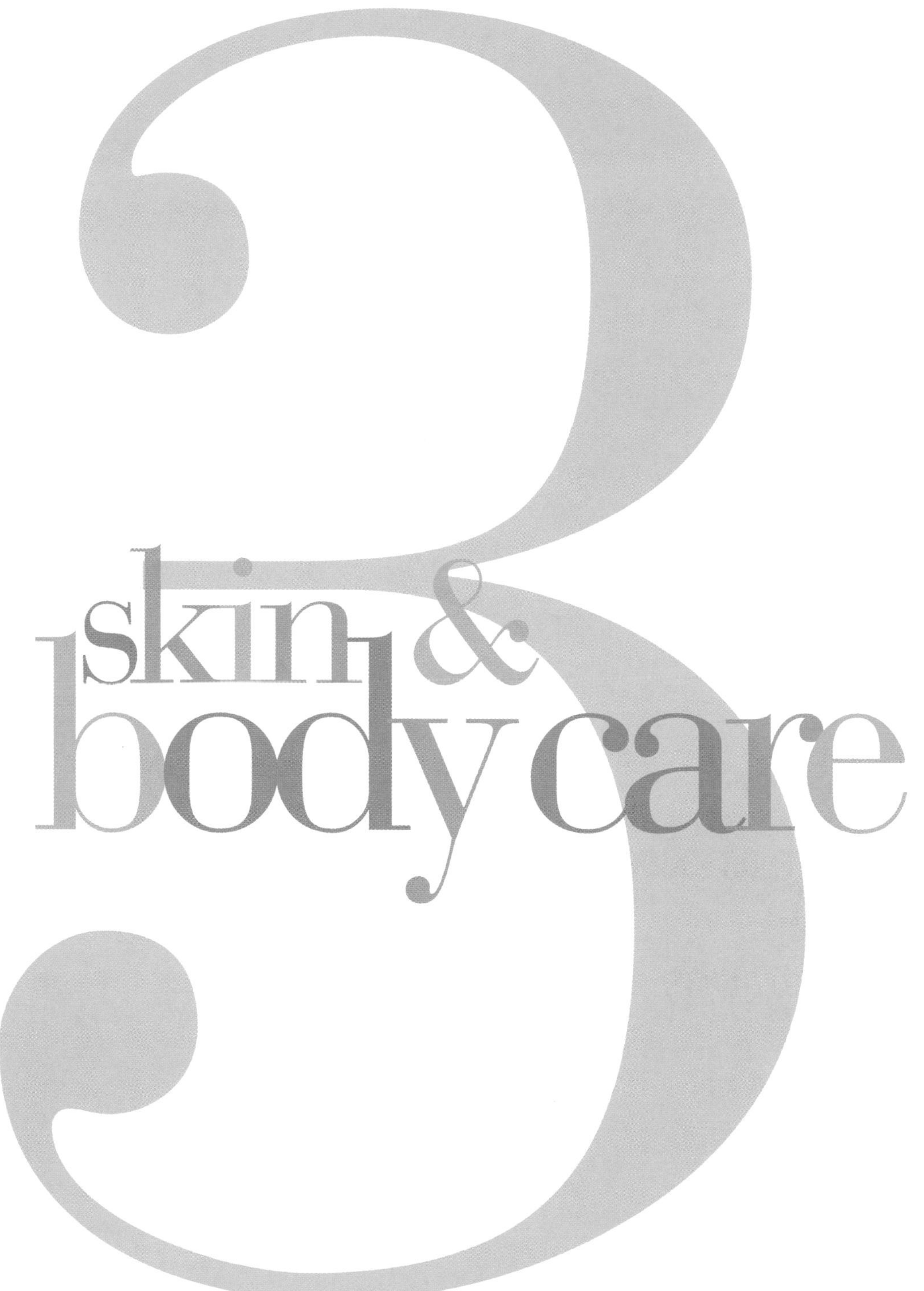

3 skin & body care

FAVORITE TREATMENTS

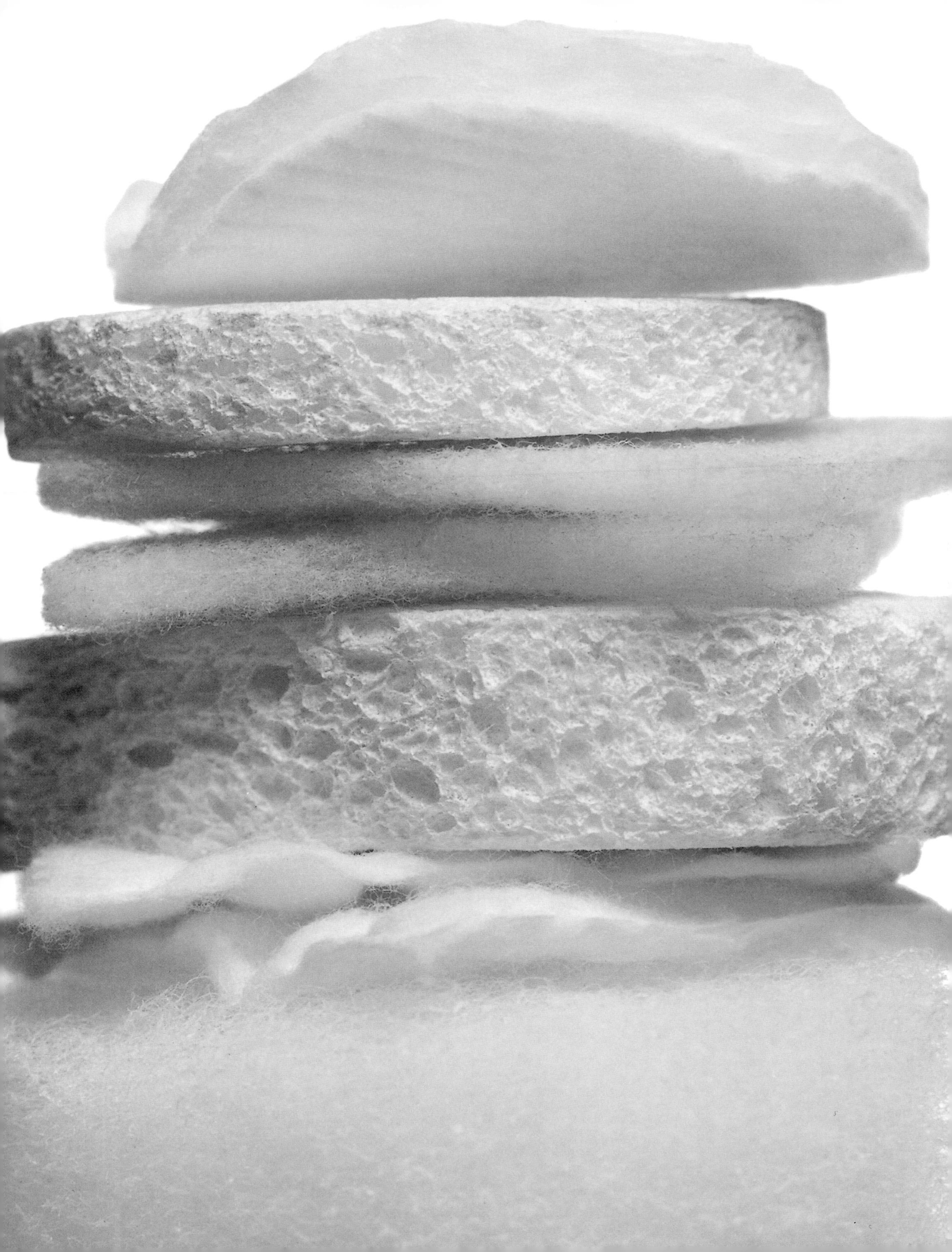

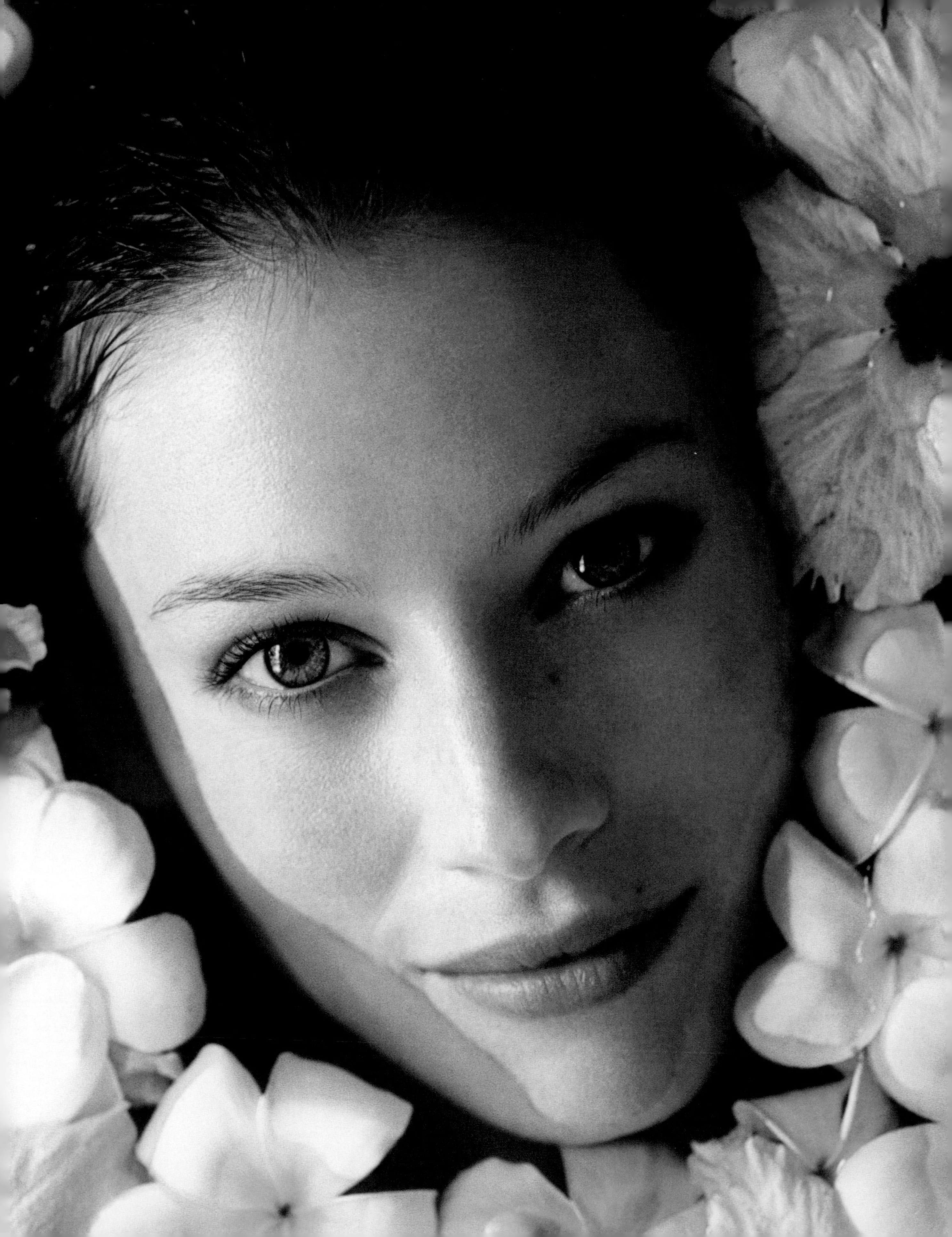

Skin care: In-your-face beauty

Menu for a fresh complexion

Start your morning off right with beautifully refreshed skin to brighten the rest of your day. Here are tips from the pros for perfect skin

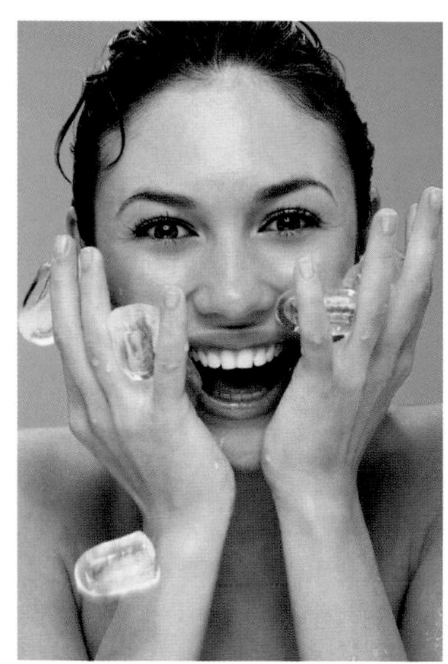

WAKE UP FRESH WITH A SPLASH OF WATER!

The only way to prepare and care for your skin before applying makeup? Routine washing to remove all the dead cells accumulated overnight in your sleep.

A generous splash of cool water wakes up your skin, then follow with 30 seconds of exfoliating to remove the traces of sleep and activate **microcirculation** on the face and neck area.

Start with warm water and gradually switch to cold. You can do a quick wash **in the shower** or a more gentle one using a cotton washcloth. In either case, dab dry with a soft, absorbent towel to prevent irritation.

Use a cotton swab dipped in lotion or in water to **clean** the corners of the eyes of any nighttime secretions, then use a small makeup remover pad to separate the lashes, prevent clumping, and remove any leftover traces of mascara.

Warm some facial cream in your hands and **massage** your face, neck, and upper chest, working from the center out. Use a light touch, especially around the eyes and mouth, moving gently. Remove any excess facial cream before applying makeup or else it won't adhere properly.

You can have **rosy cheeks** (almost) naturally: just delicately pinch your cheeks, and the pink will appear!

SECRETS OF A MAKEUP ARTIST

You should not put ice directly on your skin as seen in the photo above (it hurts!), but a bit of ice wrapped in a napkin or washcloth will do wonders for freshening up your complexion and giving it a rosy glow!

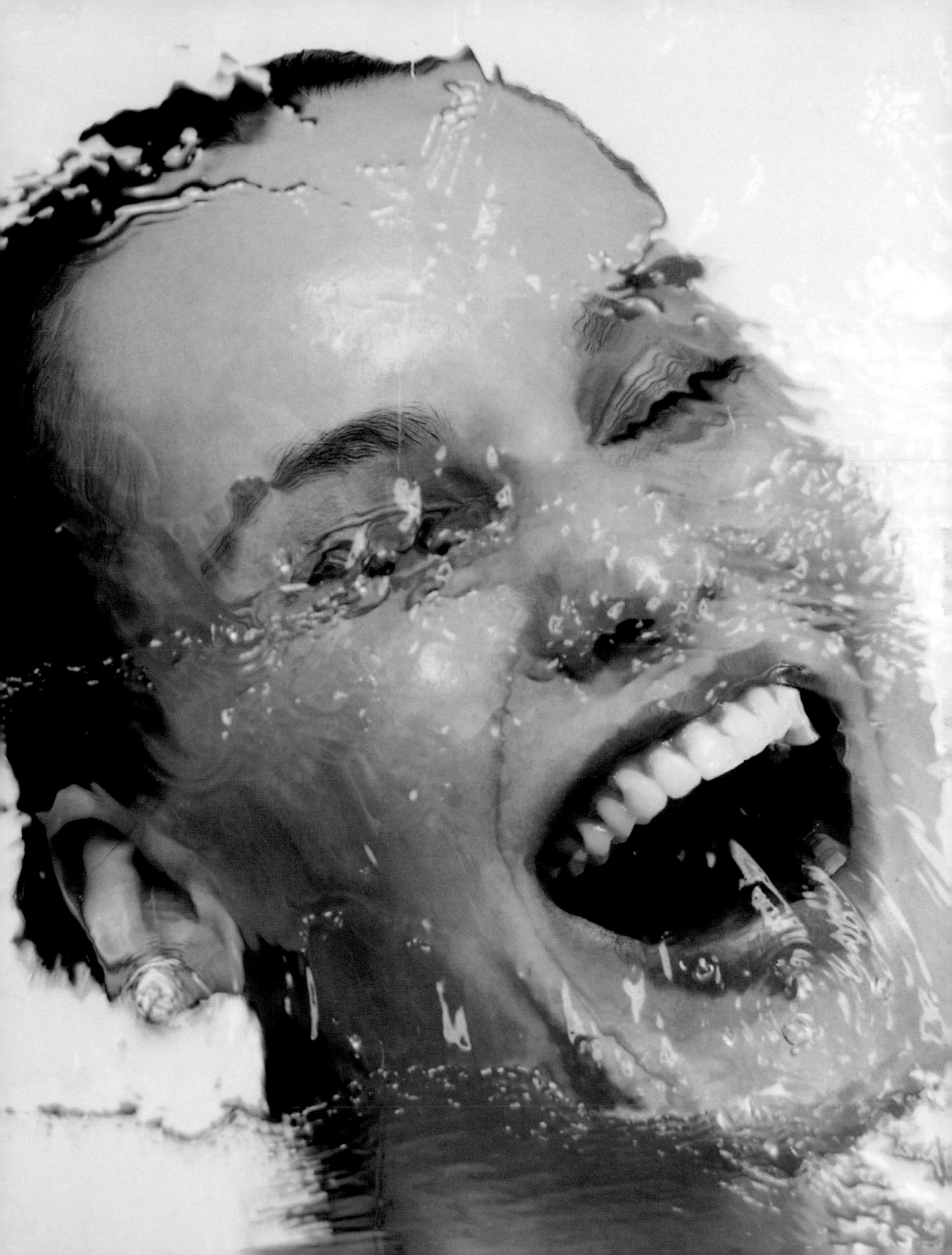

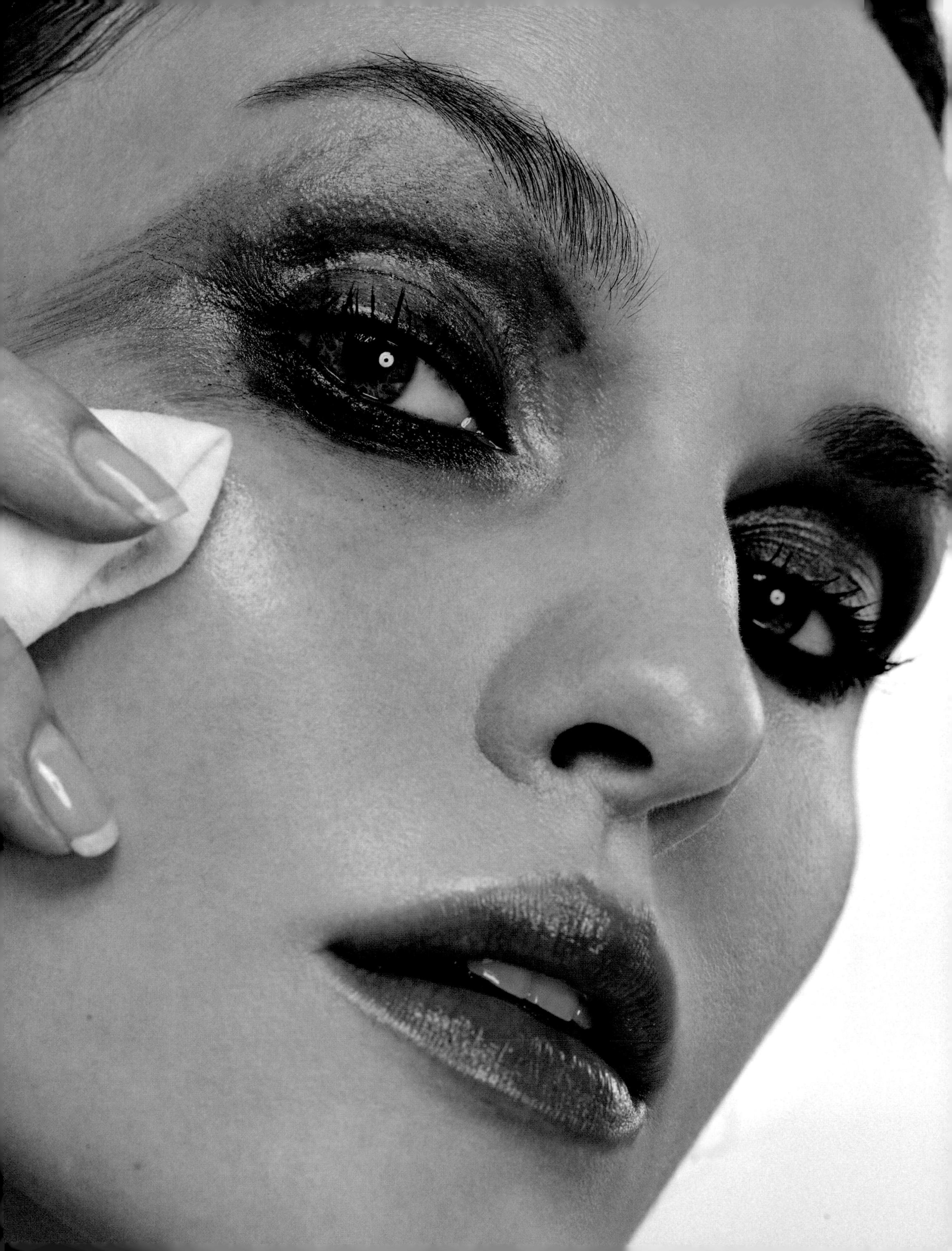

Eye care in the wink of an eye

Particularly sensitive, the skin on our eyelids truly deserves special care.

ATTENTION: FRAGILE AREA

The skin on our eyelids is extraordinarily thin and has an unimaginable complexity. It consists of no fewer than seven layers, which multiply the risks for swelling and bags. The eye rests on a small cushion of fat that has the ability to change its shape with the slightest disruption. The perpetual motion of the eye muscles results in the first wrinkles and signs of aging.

MADE TO ORDER

Specialized care products to be used around the eyes (anti-wrinkle, anti-dark shadows, anti-bags, anti-sagging), which are ophthalmologist tested and developed especially for sensitive skin, are preferred to products formulated for the rest of the face, no matter how high quality they might be. Use the same principle for makeup removal lotions and gels—many of them specify "avoid contact with eyes."

THE ART OF APPLICATION

Eye care treatments must always be used in small quantities and with a very gentle touch. Place a drop of the product on the tip of your finger and massage with a circular motion. **Anti-dark-circle and anti-bag treatments** help drain the fluid around the eye area. Use gentle pressure from the fingertips and massage from the outer corner of the eye inward to "reboot" the lymphatic system and drain the water trapped in the tissues.

REMOVING MAKEUP

Remove your contact lenses (if you wear them, of course), then place a pea-sized drop of eye makeup remover on a makeup remover pad. Gently glide it across your eye without rubbing and allow it to penetrate for a few seconds. Finally, sweep the pad upward toward your temples until there is no trace of makeup.

ADVICE FROM A DERMATOLOGIST

EYE WORKOUT: Gently pinch the skin from the eyebrow's inner corner out to the temple to stimulate the upper eyelid, which has a tendency to sag.

ADVICE FROM A MAKEUP ARTIST

Pads that are already saturated with oil-based eye makeup remover are the best choice to eliminate all traces of waterproof mascara and eyeliner.

Removing makeup perfectly

We all sometimes go to bed without removing our makeup. But this is a bit like sleeping fully dressed. Take a few minutes before bed, and your skin will thank you!

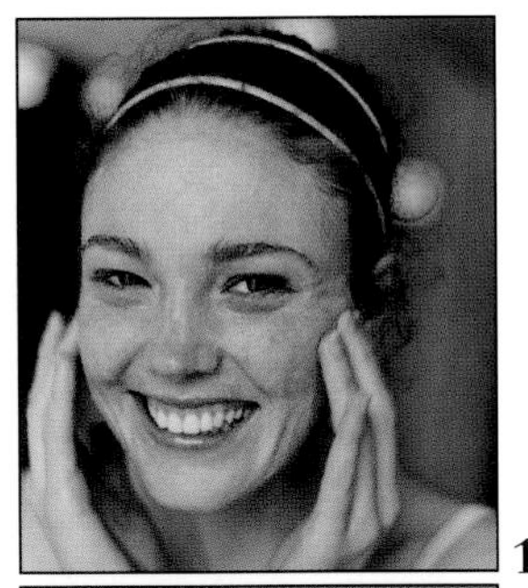

1

2

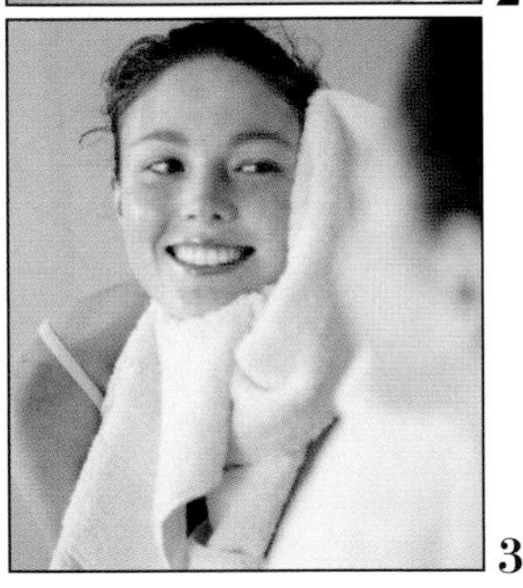

3

BEAUTIFULLY CLEAN SKIN

Before going to bed, washing your face is a true priority. All the business of the day is finished, and it's time to consciously rid yourself of all impurities, from the grime left behind by all sorts of pollution to the excess sebum from your glands, allowing your skin to finally breathe.

Without daily makeup removal before bed, excess sebum will result in the formation of pimples, **skin will suffocate,** and wrinkles will appear much sooner. And there's no use in applying night cream to a face that hasn't been properly washed first.

ALL THE FORMULATIONS

The classic duo of **cleansing milk and lotion** is but one of many different types of makeup removers that can be adapted to your skin type. Another option is a **cleansing gel or mousse,** which you apply generously and then rinse with water and pat dry gently (see photos 1, 2 and 3).

Ultrapractical are **moist facial towelettes** and **wipes** that are hypoallergenic and have the makeup remover built in.

ADVICE FROM A DERMATOLOGIST

Water can be your skin's enemy, especially if it has a tendency to be dry or sensitive. Thankfully, there are many no-rinse cleansing formulas.

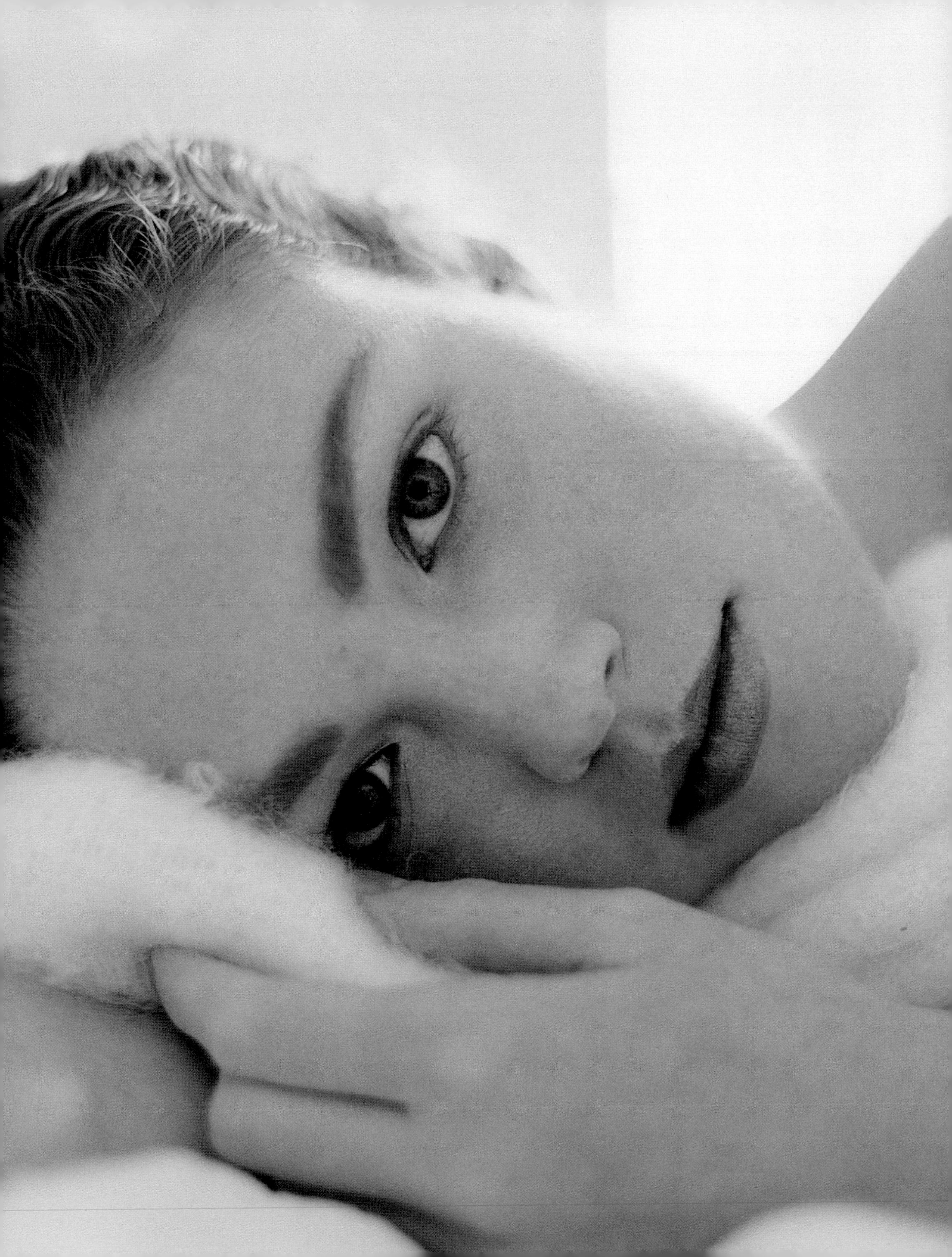

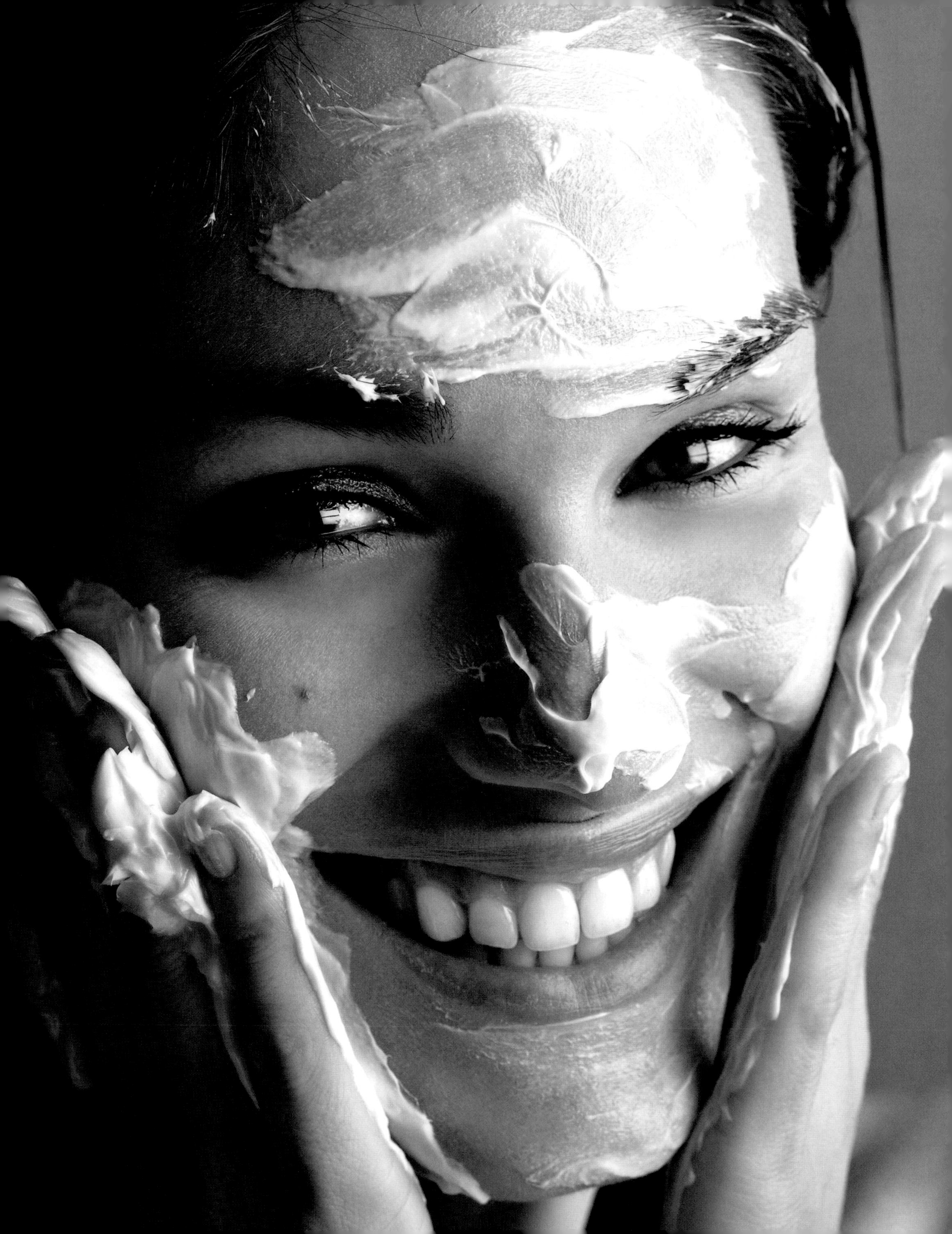

Hydration for the thirstiest skin

The water in our skin gives it suppleness and elasticity, our best beauty trait. The only problem is, water is always looking for ways to escape!

WATER FOR BEAUTY

Our skin contains about 30 percent of all the water in our body—approximately 2.5 gallons! And the daily job of skin is to try to prevent this water, which guarantees beautiful skin, from escaping. Hydration also helps us to eliminate toxins in the skin, a delicate a process that involves irrigation of all the internal layers and regulates the evaporation of superficial water. The **corneal layer** reinforces these protective devices thanks to **natural moisturizing factors (NMF),** which trap water and disperse or store it depending on the temperature.

The signs of dehydration The threshold is 13 percent water, but for normally hydrated epidermis, it's 10 percent. Dehydrated skin feels tight and lacks a healthy glow. The test: if it shows the wrinkles from your pillow when you wake up, there's no doubt that your skin is dry!

HYDRATING: CRITICAL BEAUTY RITUAL

The treatments you use must balance the evaporation of water while helping the epidermis create its hydrolipidic film and reinforce the barrier effect. Choose your skincare based on your skin type. Look for active ingredients such as glycerin, urea, and ammonium lactate.

Drink!

The guideline to follow is about 50 ounces (1.5 liters) of water per day or 68 ounces (2 liters) when the weather is hot.

ADVICE FROM A DERMATOLOGIST

STEAM:
WHY IT WORKS

Steaming your face with thermal water or mineral water not only has a deliciously refreshing effect but also contributes to mechanically reconstituting the hydrolipidic film by preventing dryness: the vaporized water, instead of water from the epidermis, will evaporate.
The water filtering through the corneal layer comes mainly from the dermis and evaporates progressively.
The phenomenon of undetected perspiration accounts for 20 percent of our daily water losses.

Daily nourishment

*Renew your skin in a few minutes.
These automatic refreshers will transform your everyday routine!*

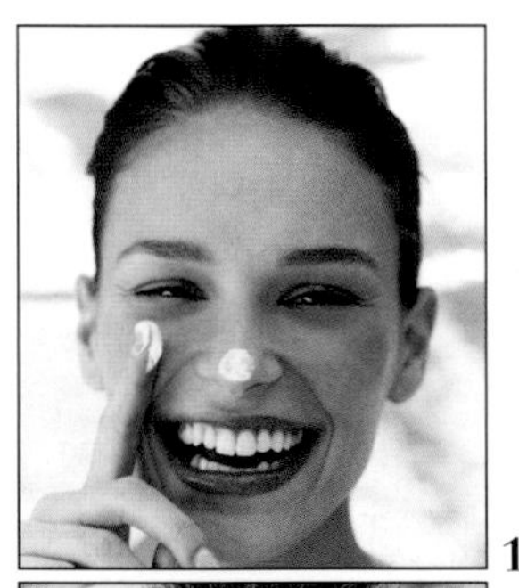

1

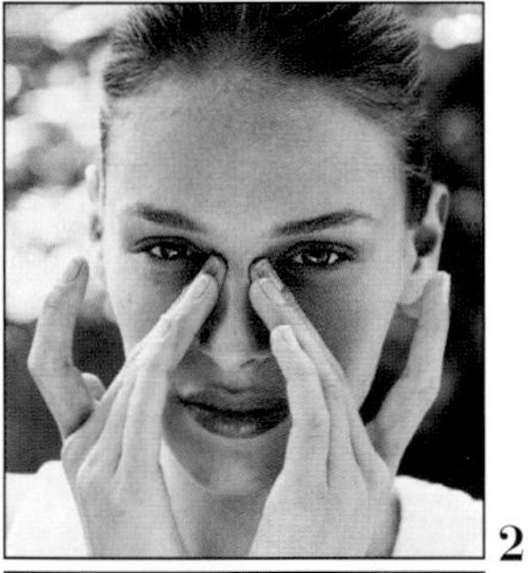

2

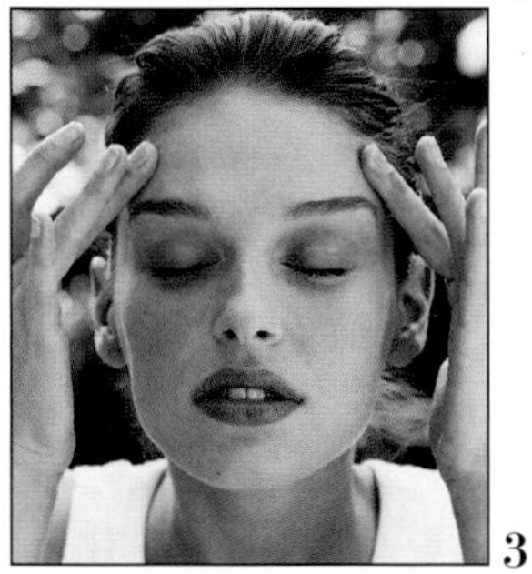

3

EXPERT CARE IN THREE EASY STEPS

1 **Choose** a good product: one with a pleasant texture and fragrance (or unscented if you prefer), and, most importantly, one that matches your skin type and its needs.

2 **Massage** the critical areas around the eyes to drain the fluid that has built up. Start from the inner corner of the eyebrow and use gentle pressure with the pads of your fingers.

3 **Smooth** the fine lines upward. Your skin will appreciate this pampering and will send the grateful messages to your brain.

Night creams work well for those whose skin has a tendency to be dry. Use rich creams with an oily texture.

Day creams are lighter formulas with more water than oil.

ADVICE FROM A MAKEUP ARTIST
Facial massage, which is extraordinarily relaxing, gently activates the microcirculation of blood and lymphatic fluids. It also reinforces the benefits of the products and creams you are applying.

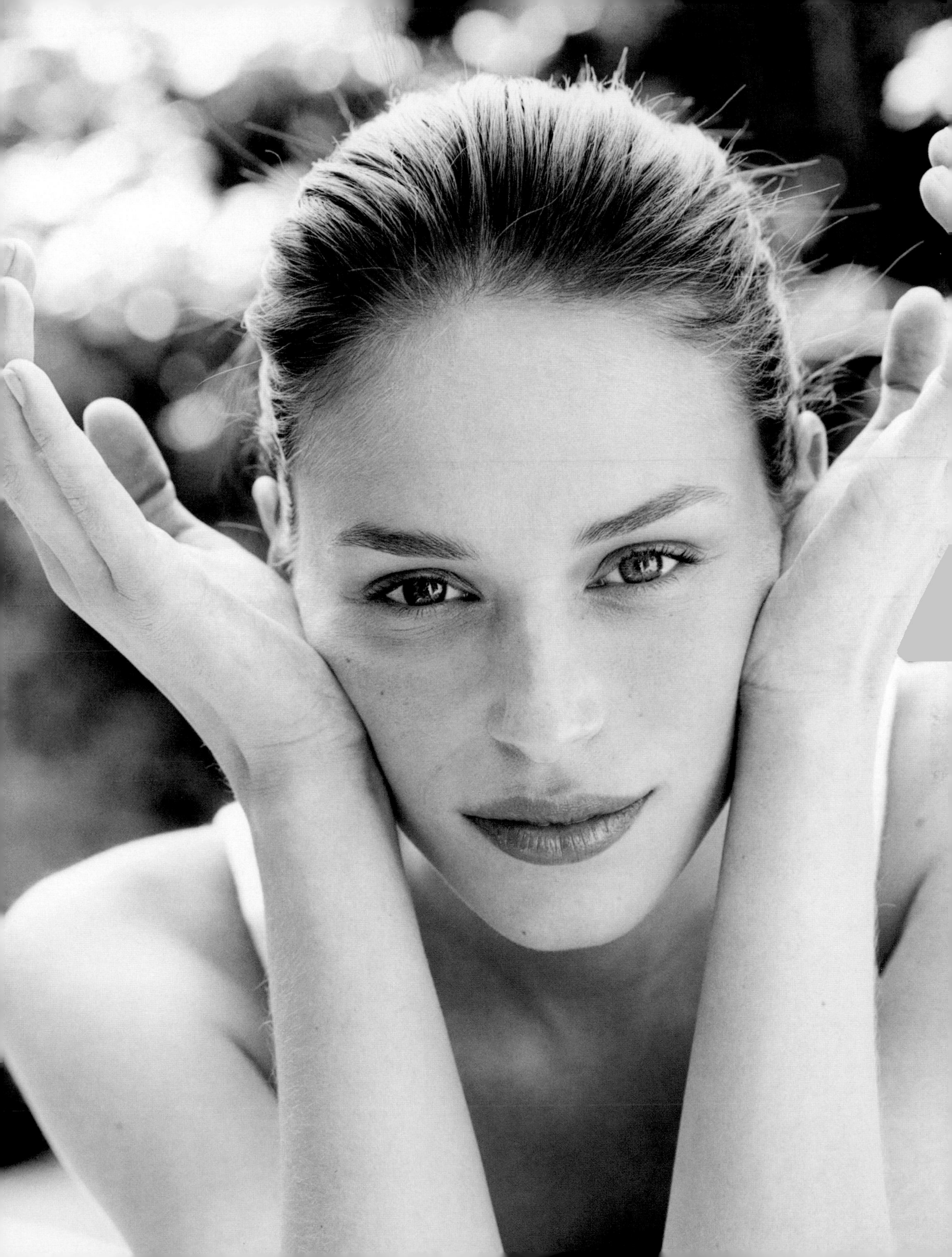

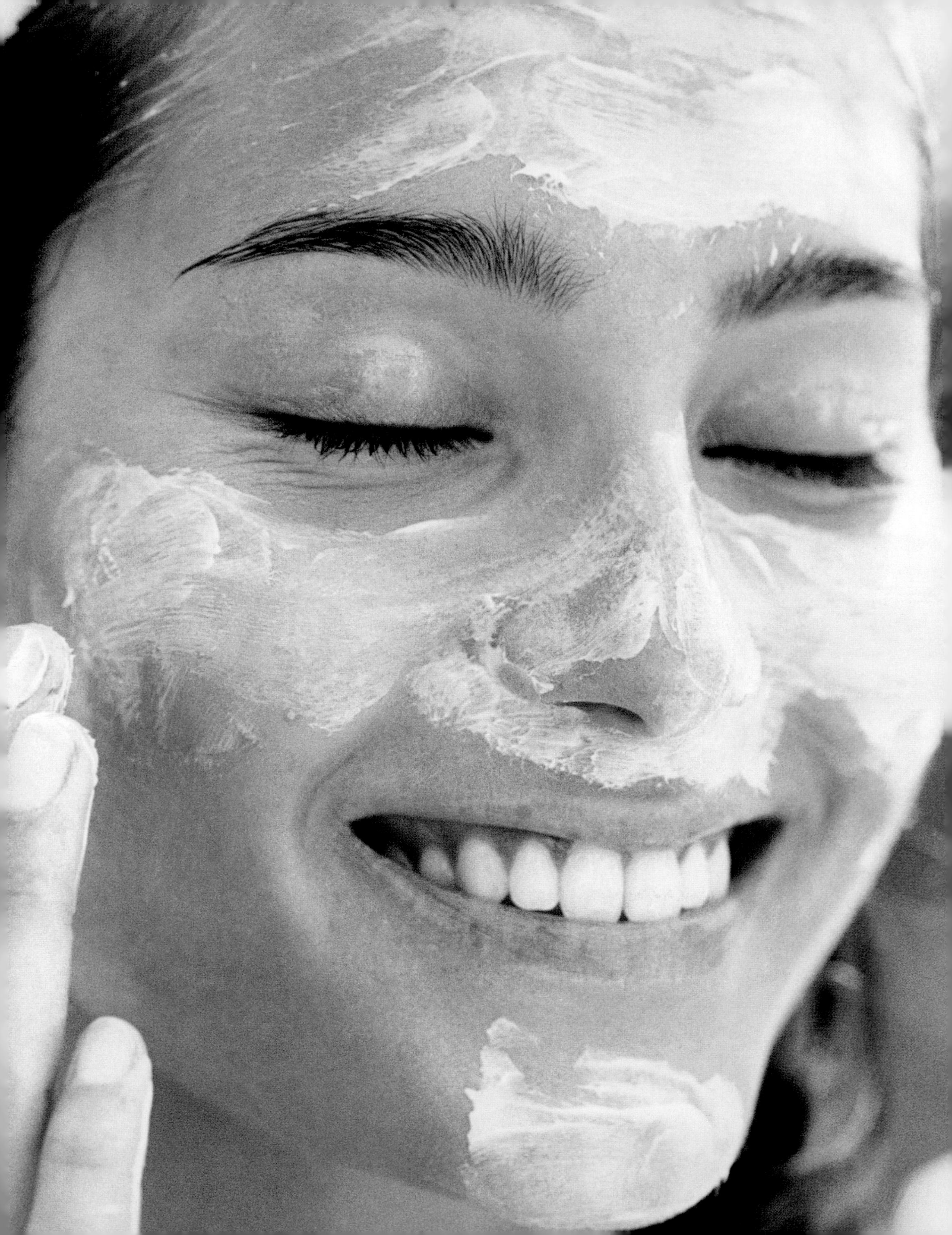

Exfoliate for a healthy glow

Do your skin a favor: deep-clean the skin with a purifying mask—it'll help make the most of your everyday skincare routine.

CRAZY FOR EXFOLIATION!

Exfoliation is the only way to renew skin without a visit to the dermatologist. With microcirculation stimulated, your skin tone is brighter, and the skin is better prepared to allow the active ingredients of your other skincare products to penetrate and take effect. Apply the exfoliant and gently massage in small circles around the lips, neck, and décolletage as well (but be sure to avoid the eye area). Make this part of your weekly routine.

CHEMICAL PEELS AND MICRODERMABRASION AT HOME

These treatments gently exfoliate your skin, offering the luxury of professional cleansing. Chemical peeling uses active fruit acids.

BEAUTIFUL MASKS

- **Cleansing:** absorbs oil and cleanses, eliminating impurities and dead skin cells
- **Oily skin regulation:** absorbs excess sebum and normalizes the acid-base balance
- **Hydrating:** moistens the skin and jump starts the process of hydration to repair the hydrolipidic film
- **Firming:** stimulates the tissues for the dilation of veins
- **Lifting:** reshapes skin with a smoothing effect using active tightening agents

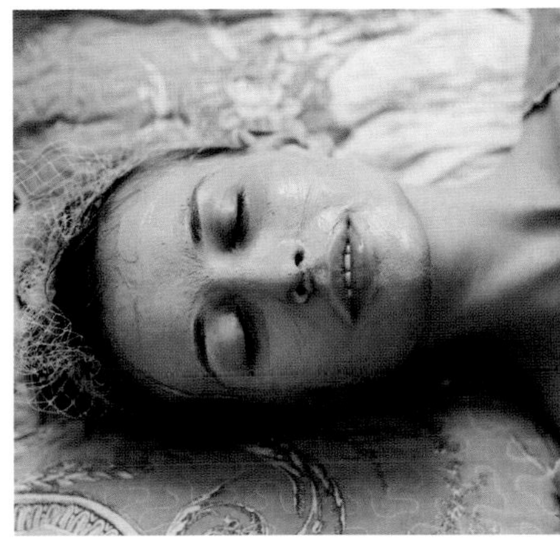

Pure clay is a classic deep-cleansing mask.

BRIGHT EYES

• Exfoliate the face with ultragentle care. • Around the eyes, buff your skin with delicate circular motion to rid your face of the dead skin cells. • Dab around your eyes with mineral water or with lotion specially formulated for the delicate skin found there. • Apply an anti-age mask designed for the fragile contours around the eyes.

ADVICE FROM A DERMATOLOGIST
Creams with a base of vitamins E and C (anti-oxidants) will brighten your skin tone.

UV rays: taming the sun

Reinforce the natural defenses in your skin so that you get only the benefits of sun exposure. Just be smart about it!

No moderation needed
A perfect partner to sun protection, self-tanners, bronzers, and beauty oils give your skin a sun-kissed glow.

ADVICE FROM A DOCTOR
The sun helps calcium absorption in bones, thanks to the synthesis of vitamin D, a vital process that prevents osteoporosis. The daily recommended amount of exposure for an adult is 15 minutes in the midday sun.

SPF INDEX—WHAT DOES IT MEAN?
- 6–14: weak
- 15–29: medium
- 30–59: high
- 60+: very high

GOLDEN RULES FOR SAFELY ENJOYING THE SUN

• **Prepare yourself** internally using melanin boosters at least 10 days before and during prolonged exposure to improve your skin's tolerance.

• **The less exposure** . . . the better. Take your time and you'll have a great tan that will last. And never sunbathe between 12 and 4 p.m. Even under a beach umbrella, you need sunglasses, a hat, and a coverup.

• **Know your skin type** (see page 19) by answering this question: do I burn before I tan? No matter what your tolerance, limit your exposure time to what your skin can handle.

• **SPF** (sun protection factor for UVB rays) indicates a sunscreen's protection level. Know what protection each level offers. A sunscreen protects not only the surface of your skin but also its chemistry (by guarding against inflammation) and its internal structure (by guarding against cellular alterations).

• **Choose a higher SPF** to get greater benefit from all the active ingredients. Sunscreens above SPF 50 are best. Also look for "broad spectrum" protection.

• **Cover your body** from head to toe with sunscreen but don't massage it in too much. The filters must remain on the surface or they can lose their effectiveness. Use high-SPF sunscreen sticks for delicate areas and **reapply every two hours**.

• **"Water resistant"** equates to two 20-minute swims spaced 15 minutes apart. If you dry off after each swim, reapply sunscreen or you'll burn and turn as red as a lobster.

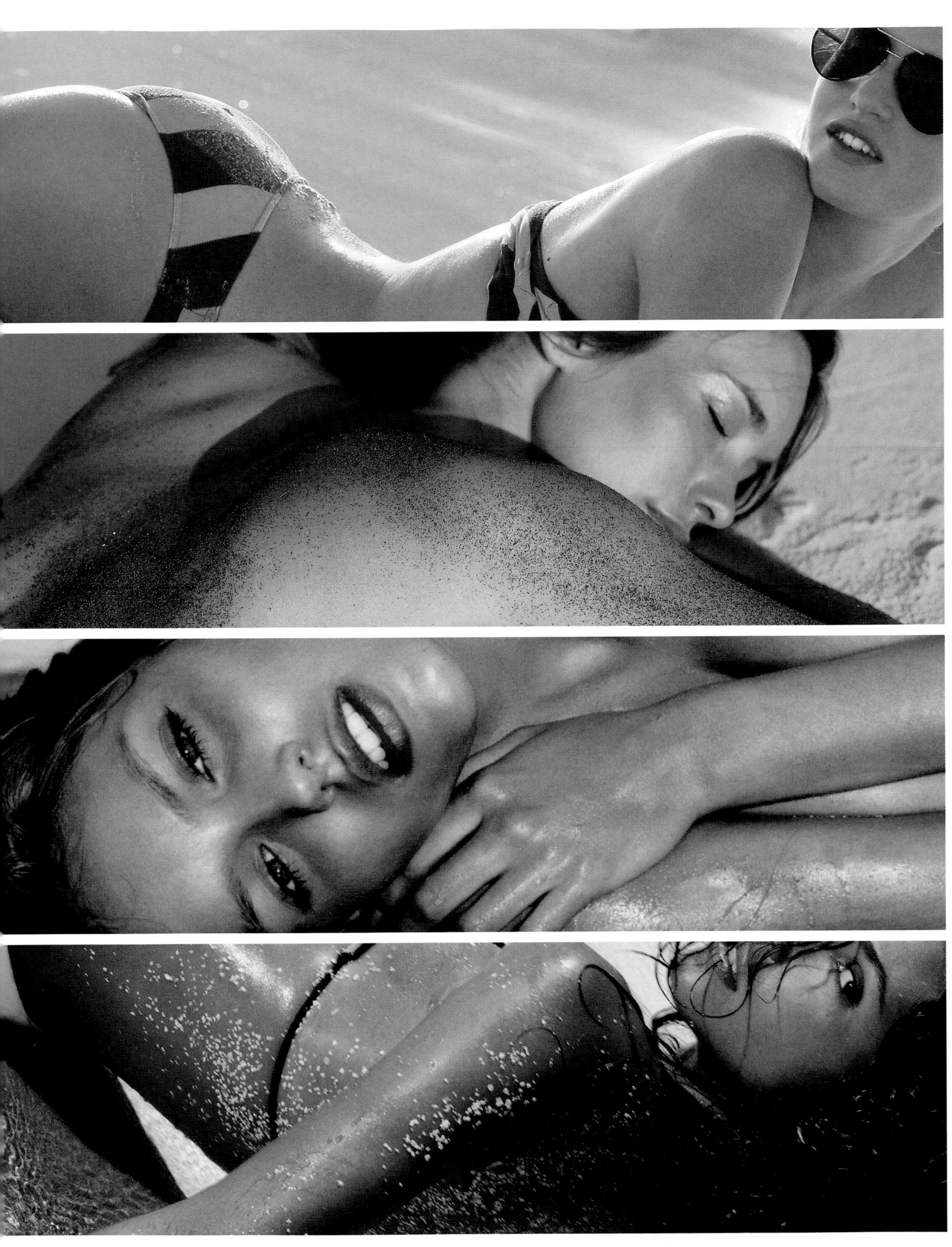

Dr. Pascale Mathelier-Fusade
Dermatologist and Allergist

Dr. Pascale Mathelier-Fusade practices medicine at the Allergy Center in the Tenon Hospital in Paris and is conducting research on sensitive and reactive skin. She is also working with Mixa cosmetics, applying her expertise as a specialist in sensitive skin to help protect the skin of women over 40.

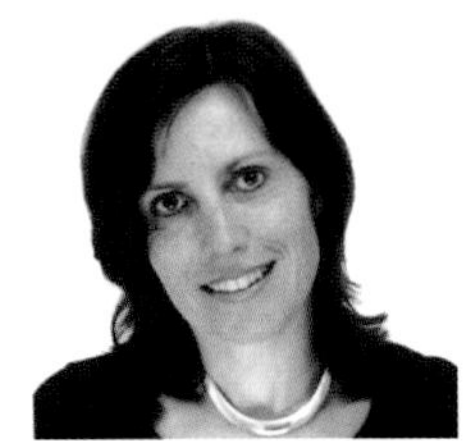

"The fact that we constantly expect our skin to adapt to risks is making it fragile!"

SENSITIVE SKIN IS GETTING MORE AND MORE SENSITIVE!

Whether it's a trend or the consequence of our environment becoming more aggressive, more and more women are declaring their skin to be sensitive. It is difficult to determine the source of the phenomenon—which we used to call "fragile skin"—because of its subjectivity. It's tough to quantify tightness, tingling, burning sensation, even if you use objective parameters. Traditionally, sensitive skin ranges from very fair skin that reddens at the slightest emotion to dry skin that seems to tolerate no cosmetics to naturally intolerant skin frequently suffering from rosacea. But among my patients, more and more have skin that was not originally sensitive but has become more fragile as a result of poorly chosen or improperly used localized treatments (antiacne medication, improper or too-frequent exfoliation). This hypersensitivity results from an alteration in the skin's barrier, the stratum corneum, the most superficial upper layer of the hydrolipidic film, which is extremely thin.

THE WORST ENEMIES OF SKIN?

Water is the worst aggressor. Whether it's hard or not, it is at the top of the list, right before detergents (**soaps, shower gels**). This is largely demonstrated by the hands, but it's also true for the face.

Climate change, sun exposure, and intense cold are also on our list of culprits. It's not just cold that's an aggressor that causes our skin to suffer but also extreme changes in temperature. When you move from cold to hot, the vessels dilate easily. On the face, where the network of veins is very delicate, redness as the result of temperature change can last a few minutes.

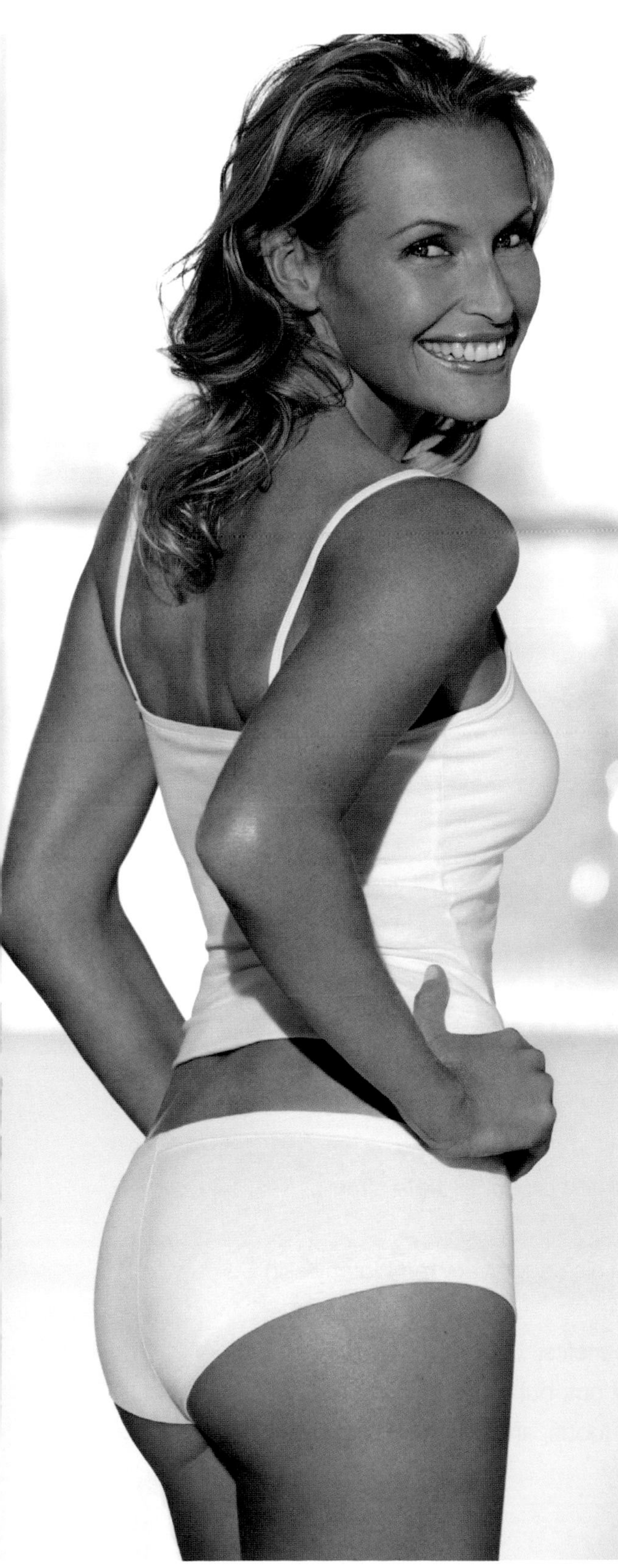

At the same time, air-conditioning has a negative impact on skin by drying it out—you also feel it in your eyes, especially if you wear contact lenses.

People with hyperreactive skin, whose nose and eyes react to all these factors, know all about it.

Pollution is obviously a problem for skin as well.

SENSITIVE SKIN: SIMPLE ANNOYANCE OR GENUINE ILLNESS?

WHEN DOES SENSITIVITY BECOME ALLERGY?

What difference does intolerance make? When a woman's skin cannot tolerate anything, when no product works for her, neither day cream nor night cream, she concludes, "I must be allergic!" But it's more complicated than that. There is a simple way to distinguish the difference between allergic and intolerant: an allergy causes itching, and skin will eventually become dry and flaky. Sensitive skin, on the other hand, will cause feelings of discomfort: burning (similar to razor burn), tingling, and stinging.

How do you test for sensitivity, and what do the results show? The results are as diverse as the subjects who are the basis of the analysis. You can tell if a product will aggravate allergies. When it comes to sensitive skin, however, the only criteria to judge are the words of the patient.

The skin is the mirror of the soul. Even if you have not clearly made the parallel between stress and sensitive skin, it has been proved that, unlike contact allergies, psoriasis and seborrheic dermatitis (which affect the scalp, the eyelashes, and the nostrils) can be triggered by bouts of stress. Of course, you can't be objective about stress, so it's very difficult to isolate the factors that set it off. What is certain, however, is that we spend our lives adapting, forging ourselves a new armor to resist these aggressions. The fact that we constantly expect our skin to adapt to risks makes it fragile. ▶

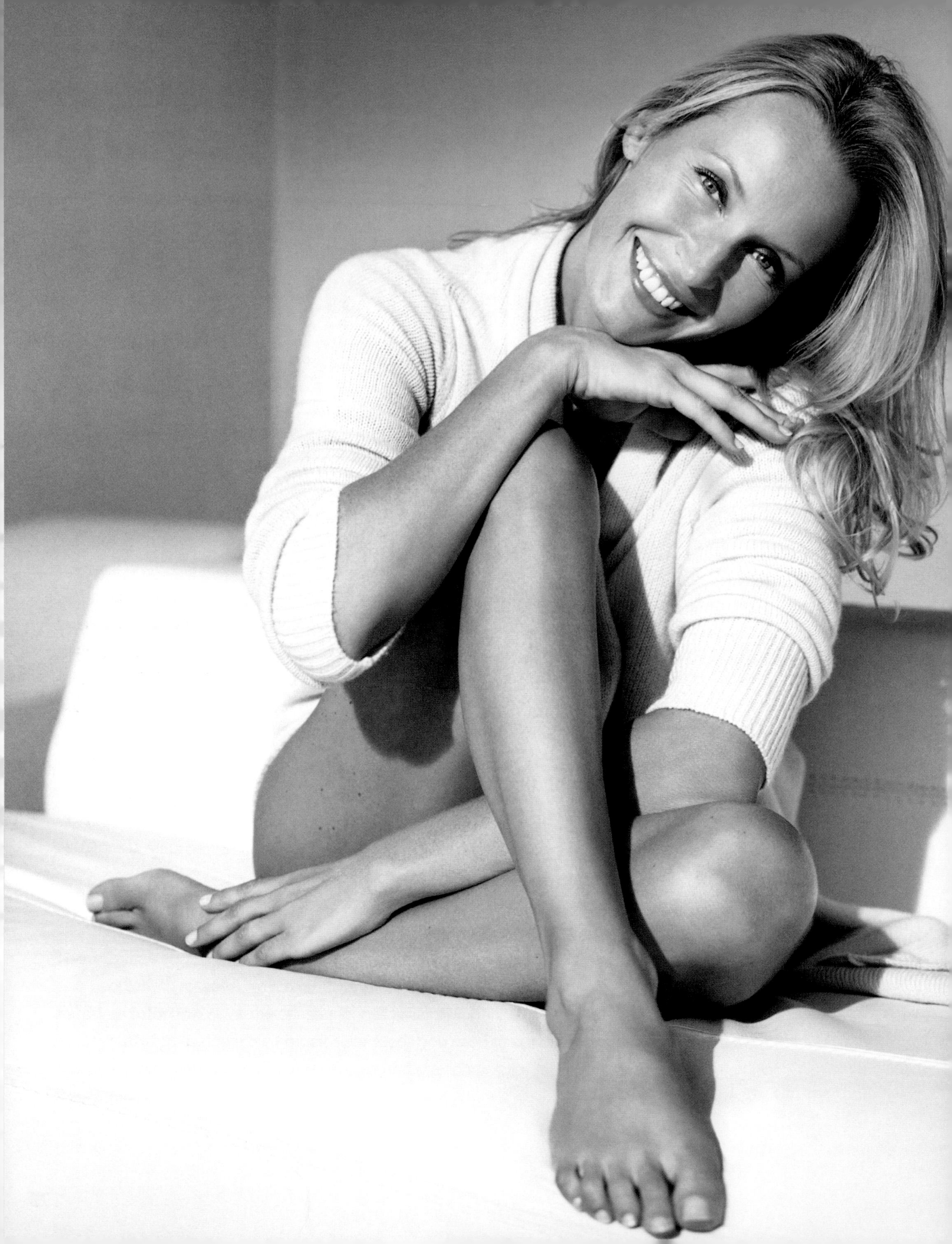

ESTELLE LEFÉBURE
TOP MODEL, ACTRESS, AND MOTHER

MY DEFINITION OF SENSITIVITY?

Sensitivity is symbolically a very strong notion with very positive elements. It's something very delicate, very gentle. You feel and are affected by everything: every movement, every word, every vibration, including those that are negative.

Nonetheless, it is important to channel this sensitivity; you absolutely must learn to cultivate it—it's a bit of innocence left over from childhood, a sort of virginity. It's very pure and something that you can lose little by little over the years.

My daughters are 10 and 12 years old, and I try to make them aware of and appreciate the simple things so that they keep their youthful innocence and don't only react to what's extraordinary.

I've been the spokesperson over the years for the organization l'Enfant Bleu - Enfance Maltraitée [a French organization protecting abused children and providing counseling for adults who were abused as children]. This is a commitment in the strongest sense, because I literally carry the voices of these children with me. It is a very sad subject that touches me more than most. It's so poignant when you see the drawings of these children. I also participate in the work being done by *Marie Claire* to educate young women and with UNICEF in Africa. There are so many causes that pull at my heart, both as a mother and as a woman. I have been so fortunate in life to be so popular and so pampered, and I find it completely natural to share this richness without expecting anything in return.

MY BEAUTY RITUALS

My beauty routine is always strongly connected with a healthy life. Everyone possesses beauty. To preserve it as best as possible, even more important than rituals and routines, there are life rules that must be respected.

My golden rule: a healthy diet, with lots of vegetables and very small amounts of meat and fish. I love green tea; it's my favorite drink; it's so healthy and full of antioxidants.

I take the time to get completely clean; **clean skin is a must for me.**

I rarely wear makeup—I'm happy to pinch my cheeks to give the impression of blush. I don't overdo it, even for evenings: a touch of lip gloss, a hint of eye shadow, a bit of mascara to bring out my lashes, since they're blonde. I never wear foundation; I simply conceal the small imperfections and brush on some powder for photos.

"My youngest daughter loves to put a dab of *cold cream* right on the middle of her cheek—it's so cute!"

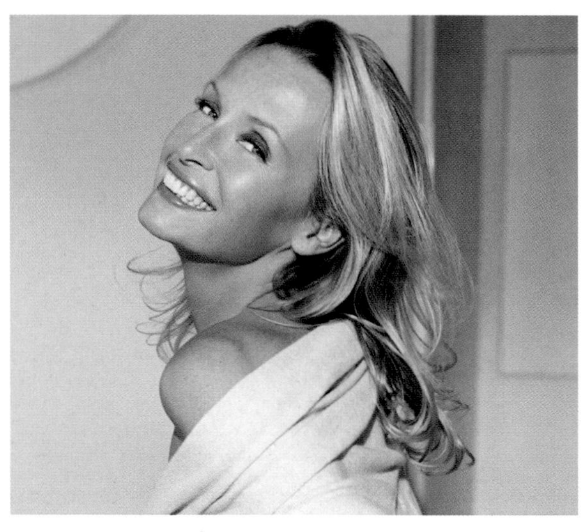

Clean skin is my top priority. And before going to bed, I have my little ritual: cream on my hands, balm on my lips, and ginger perfume. Occasionally, I'll use a hydrating or purifying mask. I make time for a massage and a more intense hydrating treatment.

SPORTY AND ACTIVE!

I do a lot of stretching at the gym. I go horseback riding and do dressage, which I love, but which is not very good for the back. It's recommended for the head, though!

I believe in many of the reflexes we learn when we're very young. I teach my daughters how to protect their skin. They love cold cream; it's so nice. They use it in the morning. My youngest puts a dab in the middle of her cheeks—it's so cute! And at least I know that, even with the cold and the pollution, her little cheeks are protected.

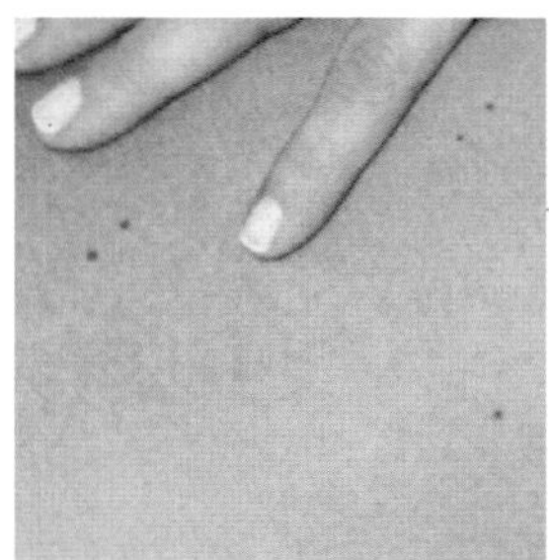

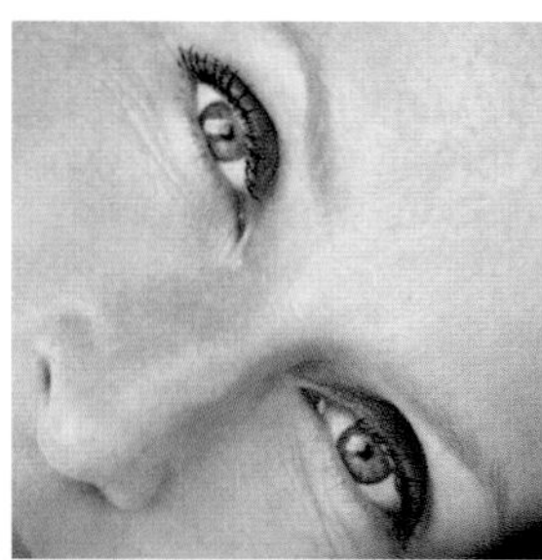

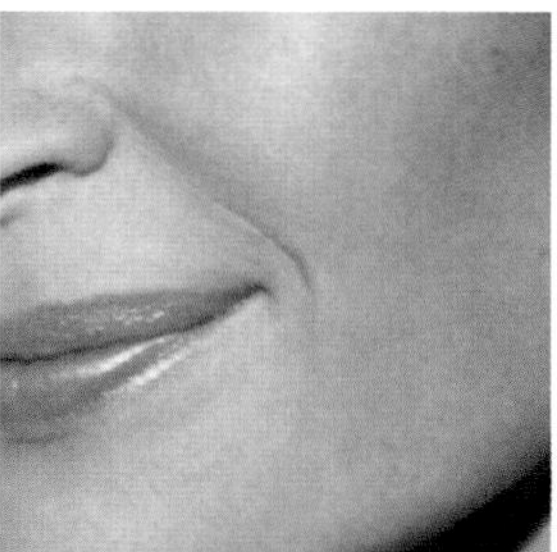

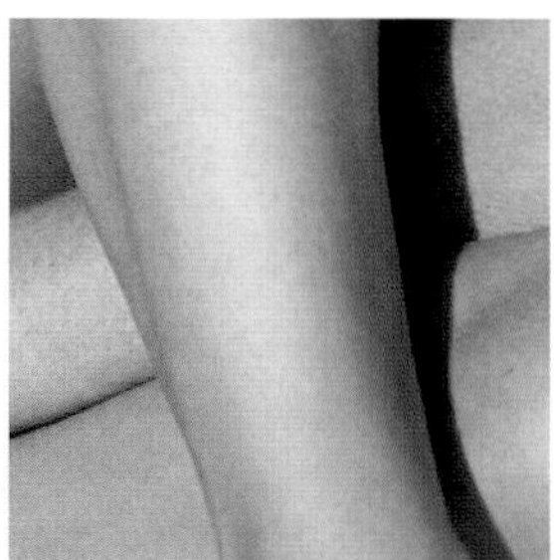

Morning and Night, Complete but gentle cleansing using a soothing makeup remover. I love the sensation of freshness, cleansing with water—and sometimes if I have a photo shoot, I'll use a cleansing lotion between two washes with water.

During the day, I'm hooked on bronzing cream, which looks great and is easy to use. And as for sunbathing and tanning, I do it very, very slowly, even though, paradoxically, my blonde skin tone gets used to it quickly.

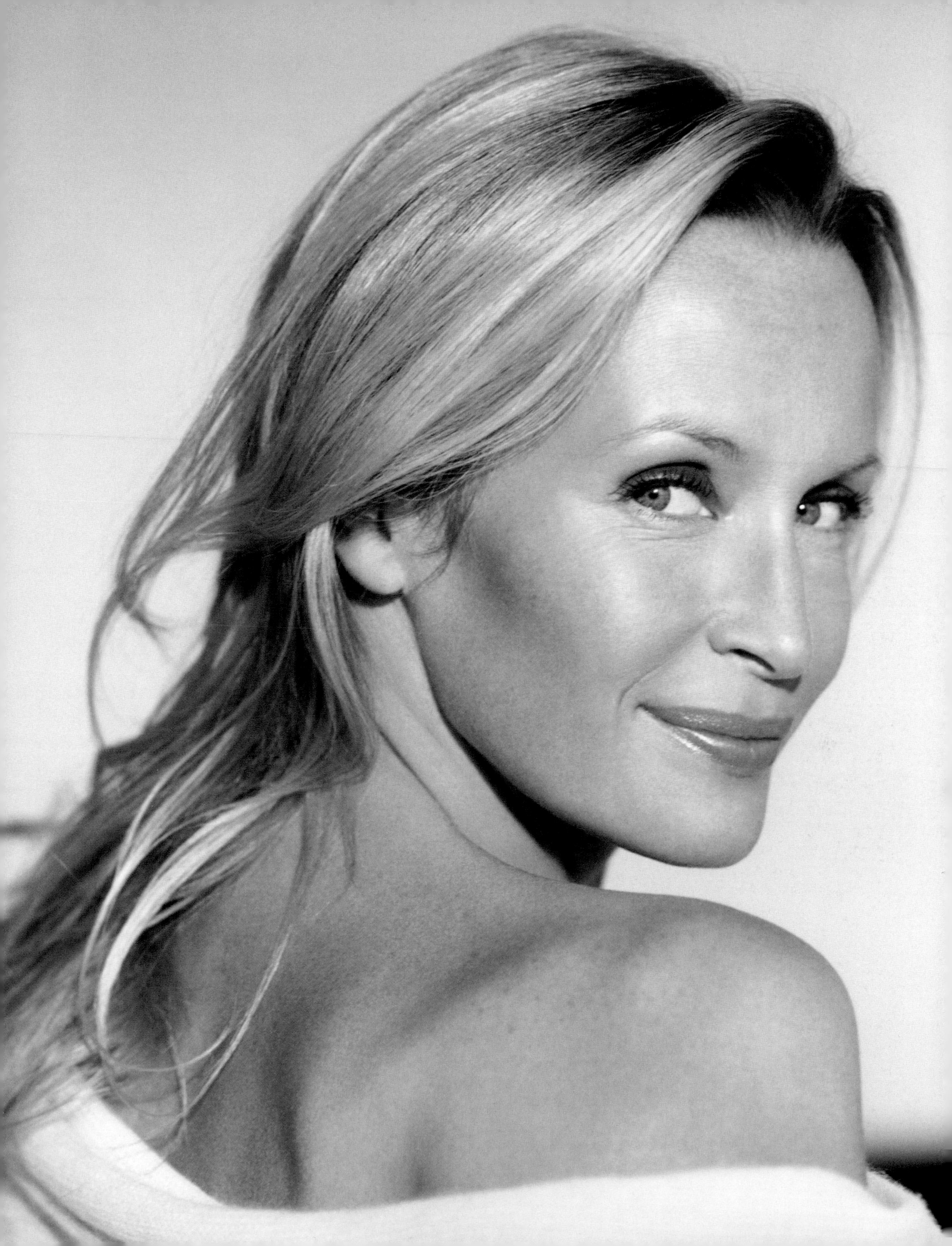

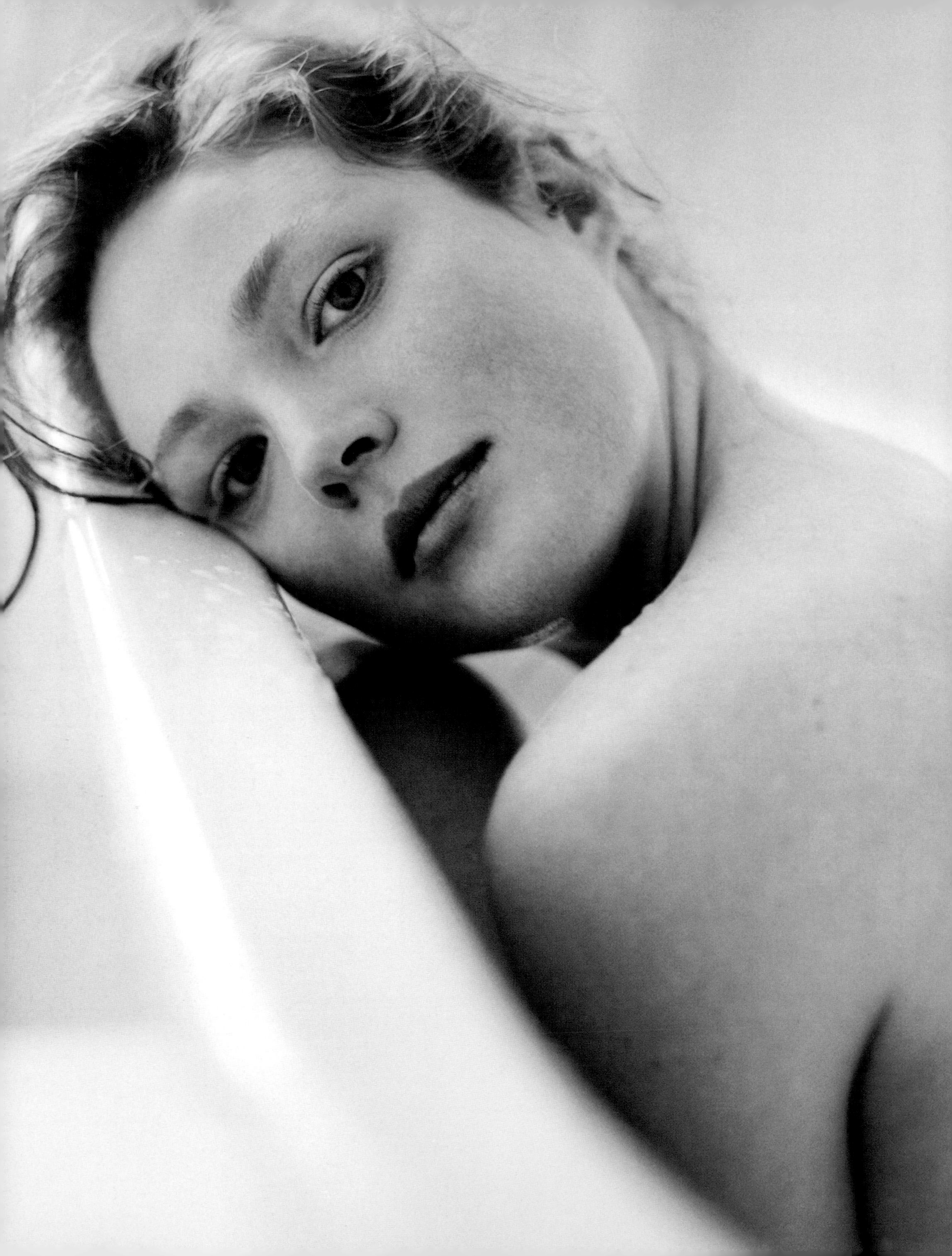

Body care: perfect harmony

Bath: dive into serenity

Like a private beach and favorite moment, a bath can be much more than just getting clean. Here's what you need to know before immersing yourself with delight.

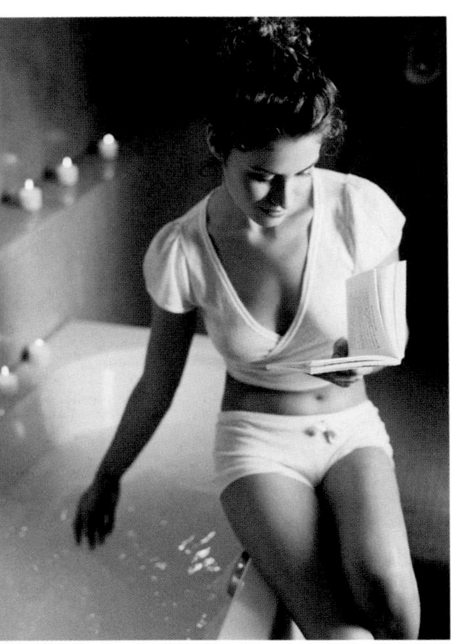

THE RIGHT TEMPERATURE

While a nice hot bath soothes aches and pains, it must not be so hot as to tire your heart or have disastrous consequences for the veins in your legs. The maximum temperature should be 99°F; however, 91°F is optimal. Always take your bath before bed (to lower your body temperature), elevate your legs out of the water (they love being raised), and, ideally, finish with a cool shower. **Essential oils** preserve the hydrolipidic film and also offer you multiple benefits from the trace elements of plants and seaweed. From relaxing to energizing, from slimming to purifying, essential oils—and the fragrance they exude—are absorbed into the pores of your skin. Bath time is also the perfect opportunity for a **beauty mask** and a **gentle exfoliation** of the knees, elbows, and feet.

TWENTY MINUTES OF WEIGHTLESSNESS

Escape the everyday routine by floating, a form of therapy that is extremely easy to practice on yourself. Get the right temperature, turn off the phone, and chase away unpleasant thoughts. Use a small inflatable pillow at the nape of your neck if the bathtub isn't comfortable enough. Keep your back loose, knees relaxed; soften your jaw and let the soothing waves and endorphins take over. Limit your bath to 20 minutes maximum so you don't wind up shivering and getting out of the bath all shriveled.

Create a retreat of relaxation with scented candles, a good book, and soft music.

To avoid any extremes, it is smart to set the thermostat of your hot water heater at 130°F.

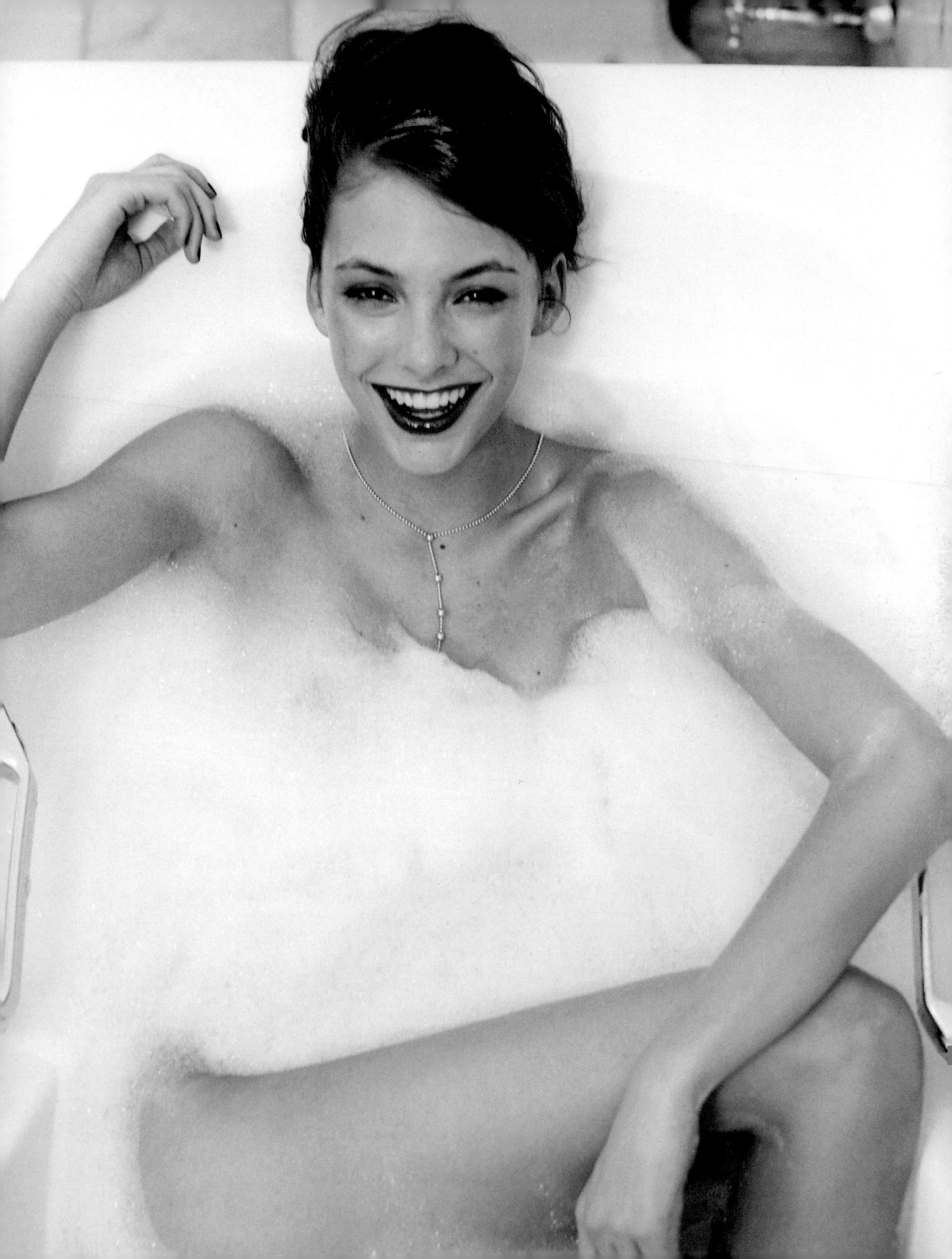

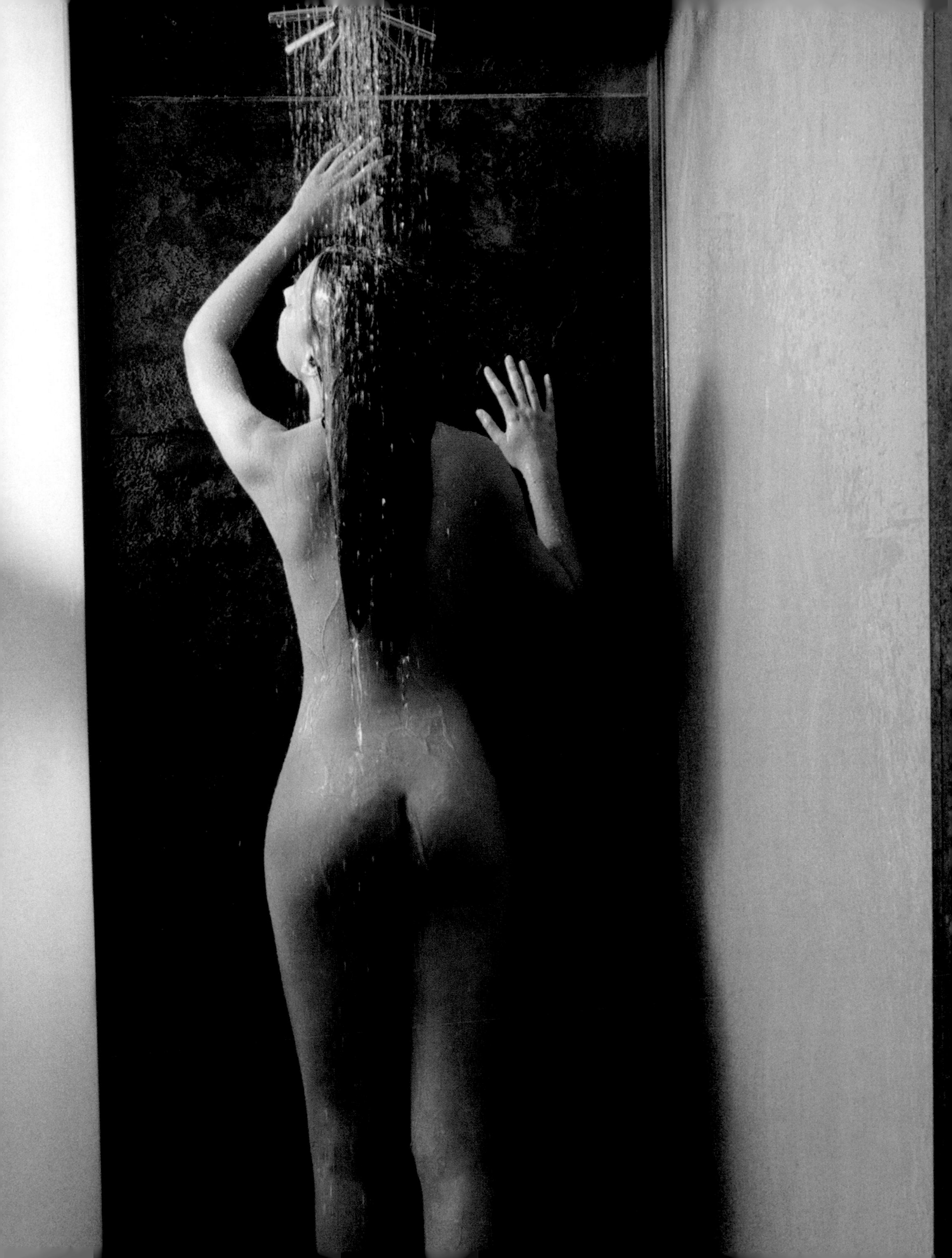

Energizing showers

An excellent tonic, a shower can wake you up in the morning, clarify your ideas, and erase fatigue and tension. And most of all, there's no better way to wash!

MORNING. . . ENERGY BONUS!

This is a great way to get rid of cramps, backaches, or any tension or tightness from sleeping in an uncomfortable position. Well-directed jets of water will massage and loosen muscles and perk you up to restart your system after being held in night's grasp.

EVENING

Summer Wash away perspiration, sand, and salt after a day at the beach or hiking, or the film from a scorching hot day in the city. Particularly beneficial and relaxing, an evening shower in the summer allows your body to forget the heat of the day and relieves the legs (as long as you finish your shower with cold water).

Winter Remove pollution and fatigue accumulated over the day. A shower allows you to recharge your batteries before an evening party. Avoid showers that are too hot since they will make falling asleep difficult.

COMFORT AFTER SPORTS

A post-workout shower eliminates the knots in your muscles and the sweat of your exertion, as well as the chlorine from the pool.

AT-HOME HYDROTHERAPY

Multiple massaging jets, Turkish steam bath, the imagination of spa designers—the possibilities are endless! The bathroom is becoming more and more a living space in its own right.

A shower uses 16 gallons of water compared to 40 for a deep bath, making it the ecological choice —except, of course, if you stand under the shower for 20 minutes.

Scottish shower is the name for the technique of starting your shower with hot water and then moving to cold. It actually comes from the hydrotherapy practices of the Scots in the 19th century.

ADVICE FROM A DERMATOLOGIST

A shower washes but also dries out your skin. Nourishing body oils and gels are an absolute must before using hydrating creams and lotions.

Erase age and fatigue

Exfoliating to reveal new skin is the survival reflex of our skin cells. It's an essential part of your skin regimen.

THE PROS

Not only does it **improve the texture** of your skin, but exfoliation also offers a perfect entrée for the active elements in the products applied (slimming, relaxing, nourishing, hydrating) since they are **more effective** on more permeable skin.

ATTACK FROM ABOVE

Use a generous dose of exfoliating scrub for the **shoulders** and **arms** and massage into your skin using a circular motion. Use the product on the backs of your arms and especially on your **elbows,** key areas that easily become dry and take on an unattractive rough look. Be gentle around your décolletage, but don't neglect it, and be especially gentle on your breasts, which should be included in the routine as well.

For Satiny Legs, start at your **ankles** and work up your **calves** (perfect for after hair removal), paying close attention to your **knees** and then your **thighs** and **buttocks,** always massaging in small circles for incredible softness.

WHEN?

Ideally, once a week (and never more than twice or you'll risk damaging the epidermis) in the shower to benefit from the moisture on your skin. And be sure to rinse fully to remove every trace of the grains from the exfoliating scrub.

ADVICE FROM A DERMATOLOGIST

A scrub or exfoliant is an extremely effective addition to your skin care routine. The tiny sanding grains are suspended in a cream that provides all the necessary softness. There are many different special body formulas, which produce different results specific to their function and active ingredients.

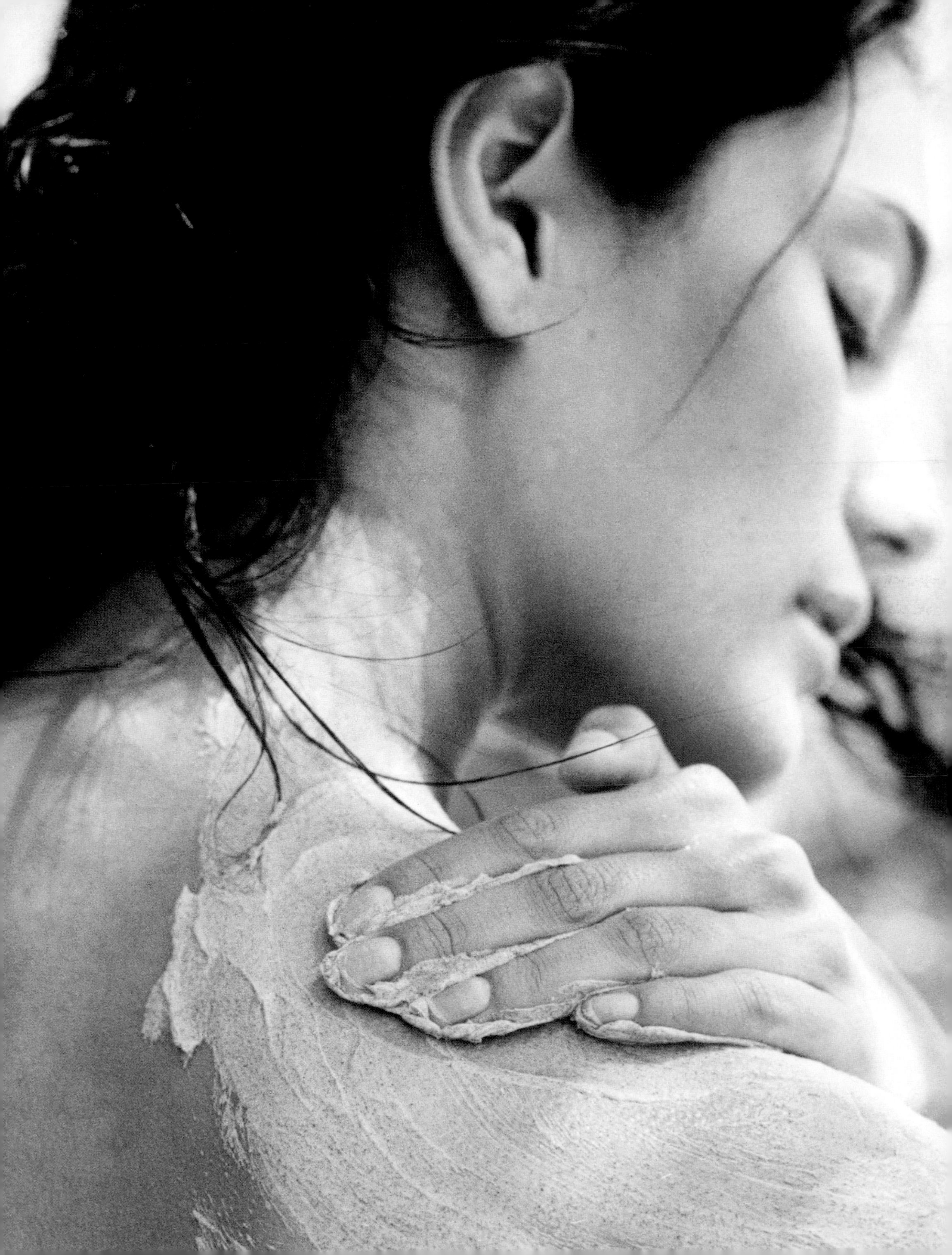

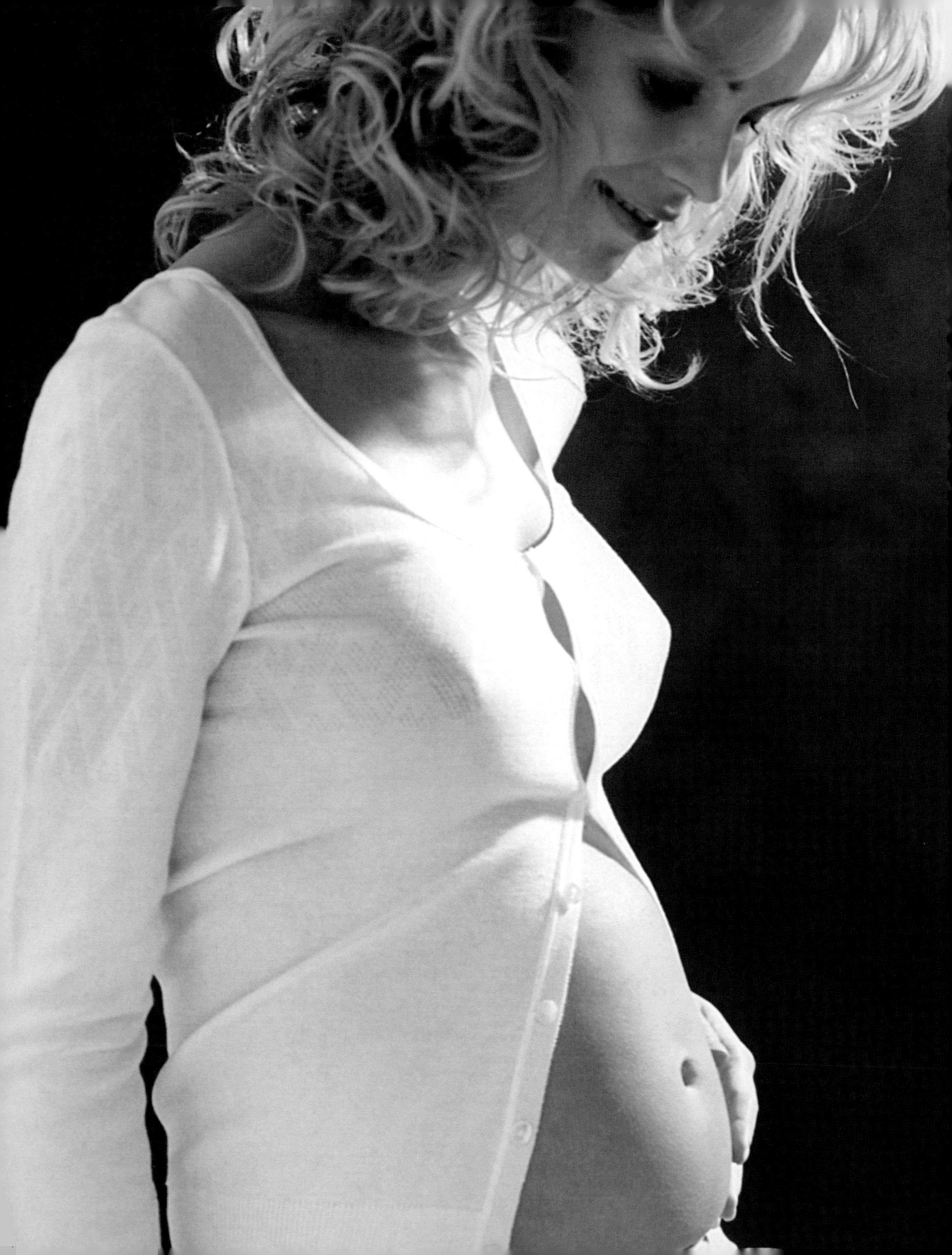

Beautiful mothers-to-be

Pregnancy is an incredible physiological digression, a serene journey that fulfills us but often leaves our skin in need of some extra pampering. Here's the user's guide.

With 100,000 times more hormones your skin is engorged with water and stocked with salt at the level of the dermis. All this ultrahydration translates into an incredible glow! Estrogen also joins the mix, meaning excess seborrhea and acne will disappear in 99% of cases.

Preventing Stretchmarks The fibers of the skin, which undergo an extreme amount of pressure during pregnancy, can crack in certain women in the layer of dermis where collagen and elastin are found. The only solution is to hydrate your belly, breasts, hips, and upper thighs frequently, at the very least in the morning and evening. Ultranourishing, these special anti-stretchmark formulas capture water molecules.

Pregnancy Mask Because the synthesis of melanin is increased, you need a total sunscreen with good protection—no exceptions!

Weight Gain must be limited and controlled. Although a large number of problems can be corrected after the baby is born, it's much better if your skin is not overstretched. Superficial cellulite (which makes your skin look like orange peel) also results from important hormonal increases. During pregnancy, the battle is a bit unequal. Drink plenty of water, avoid salty foods, and practice massage to help drain excess fluid.

Remain Firm...But Gentle Here are some recommended activities (always wear a bra!): **walking, swimming, gentle workouts, yoga, stretching, water exercise,** and **biking.**

One week before the big day, get a haircut, manicure, and pedicure.

Your hospital bag should include dry shampoo; hydrating baby wipes; gentle, unscented deodorant; mineral water spray; bronzing powder to brighten your skin; and waterproof mascara.

ADVICE FROM A DOCTOR

- Be aware that 20% of varicose veins appear during your first pregnancy, and 40% during the second.
- Being more or less prone to varicose veins is hereditary. Does your mom have them? Chances are you will, too. But perhaps your main genetic makeup comes from your father!

At the heart of hydration

Daily attention to the body is as important as attention to the face. Restoring the balance of water in the skin is a vital priority for your health.

WE MUST PROTECT OURSELVES

Our skin is impermeable to water. Otherwise, we couldn't take a bath without turning into a giant sponge! But the water that we drink every day, along with the water found in our food, continuously escapes through perspiration. That's why we must invent ways to naturally preserve it and reinforce our mechanisms of passive defense.

HELP, I'VE FORGOTTEN!

Aside from summer, when visiting the beach requires it, we have a tendency to neglect hydrating our body to protect it from its many aggressors (at the top of the list is water but also variations in temperature, the effects of the sun, and stress).

COLD DEHYDRATES . . . AND SO DOES THE HEAT!

The skin on our legs and arms, which are particularly lacking in sebaceous glands, especially suffers in winter. We protect our body with warm clothes, but we must also offer our skin a "wardrobe" of specialized treatments.

Daily use of a nourishing and hydrating cream helps the skin to reinforce its protection. This protective microlayer is comparable to sebum, forming a thin layer of hydrolipidic film through which the water in our skin cannot escape.

Water to the rescue! If you plunge yourself into a bath of water up to your chin, even if you are totally dehydrated, you will lose all sensation of thirst!

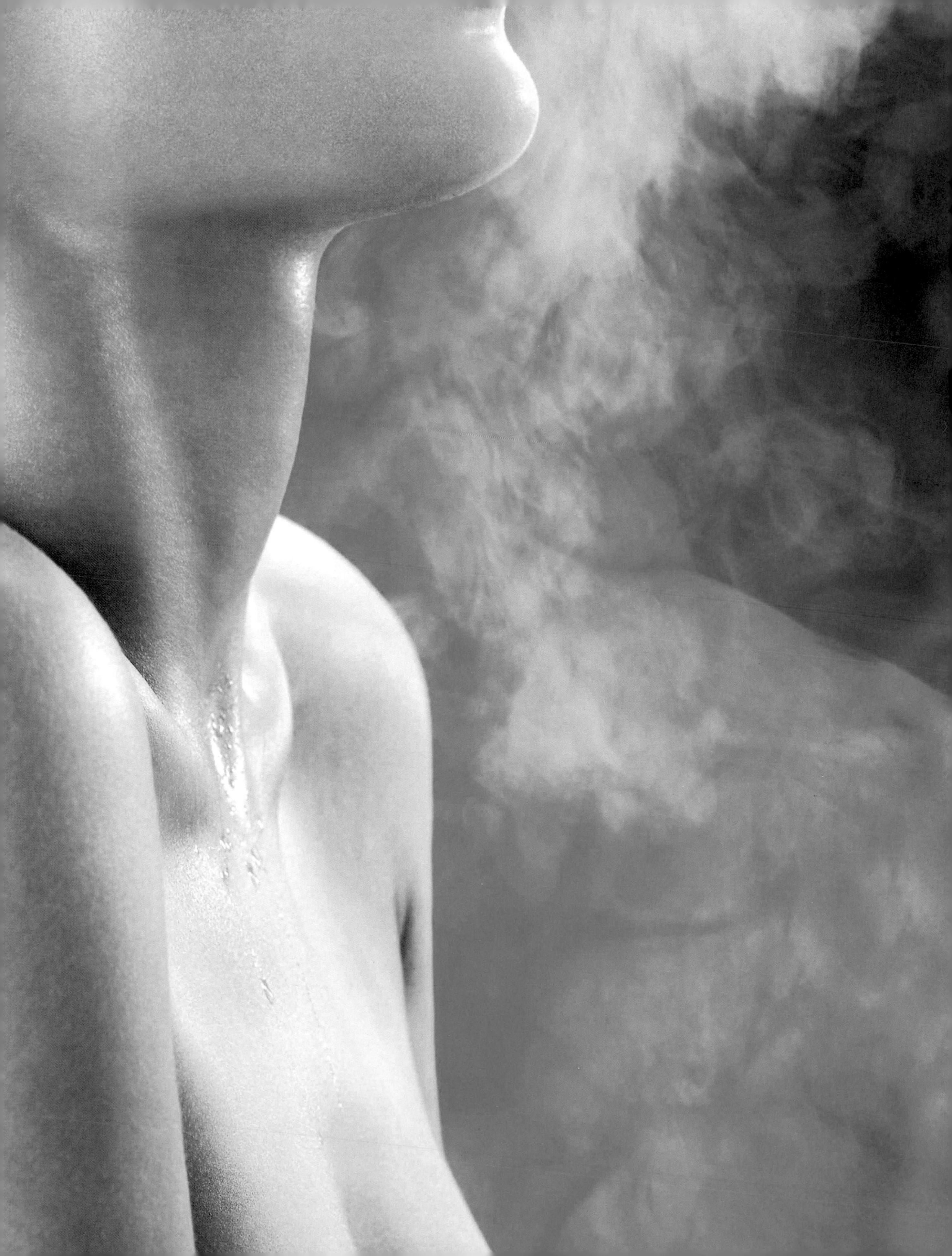

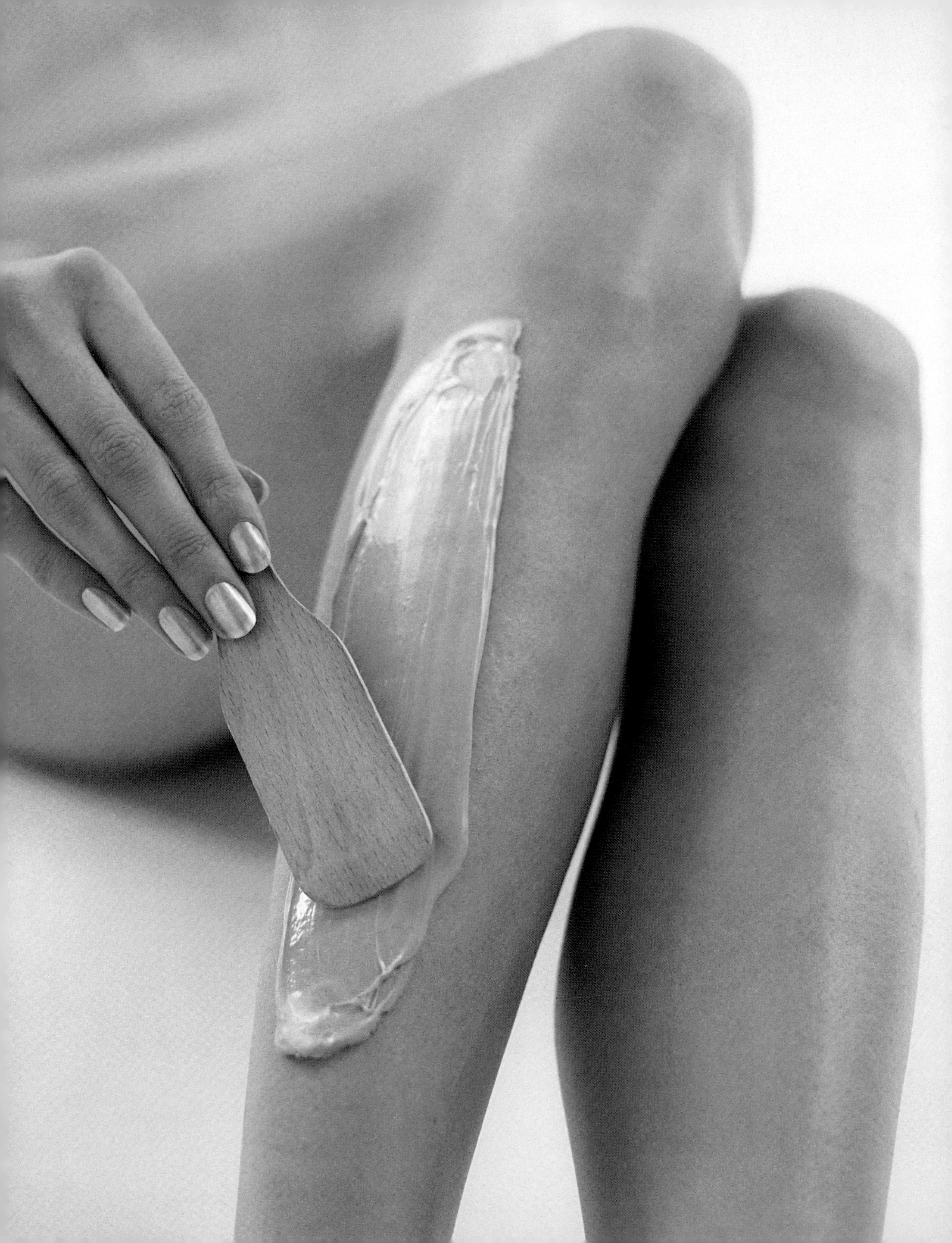

Hair removal 101

You can have the satiny legs, underarms, and bikini line that you love. You've just found the answers for smooth, hair-free skin.

WAX is the hands-down winner for longevity and effectiveness, and recent advances in softer textures make it less painful. Doing it at a salon or spa is the best way to ensure a complete job (the backs of the legs are very difficult to do on your own). There are two rules to follow: insist upon disposable, single-use wax (for hygienic reasons) and apply it warm (to avoid problems with your veins). Applying talc after removing the strip of wax will prevent irritation. To avoid ingrown hairs, exfoliate before your appointment (but never with an abrasive glove) and frequently hydrate afterward with a special cream to prevent regrowth. Use **tweezers** to remove any stray hairs. The Turkish sugaring method is an Eastern delight using honey and sugar.

A RAZOR is perfectly legitimate for emergencies. But because it cuts the hair at skin level, it does not discourage regrowth. And, of course, it can hurt! To make it less painful, use shaving creams or mousses with softeners, and always use a woman's razor. Finally, take advantage of a bath before shaving for the best-prepared skin.

DEPILATORY LOTION should be used with caution and only after testing on a small patch of skin (wait 24 hours to see the results). Rinse this off in the shower without using soap to prevent irritation.

ELECTRIC EPILATORS provide an interesting alternative to shaving because they pull out part of the root of the hair. They're much more pleasant when used with cold anesthetizing gels that are now available; it feels like an ice cube being rubbed over your skin.

BLEACHING works best for the face and arms, except in extreme cases.

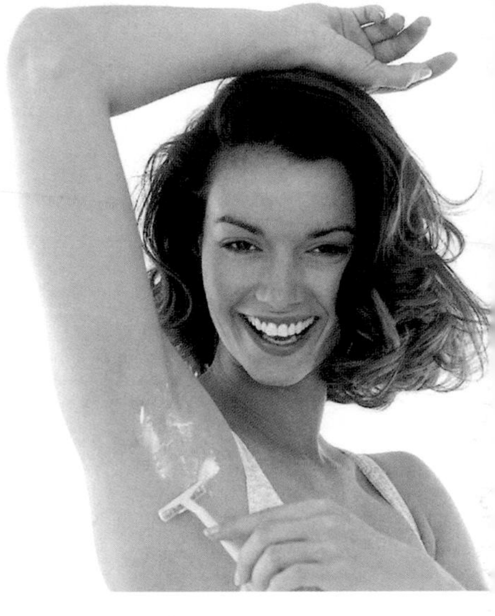

ADVICE FROM A COSMETIC SURGEON

For long-term hair removal (we no longer call it "permanent"), laser treatment uses intense pulsating light that penetrates the melanin of the hair and destroys the root. More effective and less painful on pigmented hair than previous generations, it still remains a time-consuming job that requires several months. Annual follow-up visits are also needed.

What product should YOU use?

How do you choose the perfect product from among the profusion of pots, jars, and bottles? Here is a quick guide to the textures, so you can make the most of what's available.

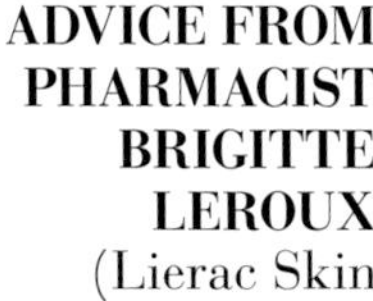

ADVICE FROM PHARMACIST BRIGITTE LEROUX (Lierac Skin Care)

Be patient: it takes 21 to 40 days (the life cycle of cellular renewal) to measure the effectiveness of a skin care product. Ineffectiveness is often connected to improper use! The multitude of different product textures available is not a marketing gimmick, and they're not interchangeable. For example, with sun protection products, even with the same SPF, a cream might be better in terms of coverage than a spray.

MASKS

These are the pros of home skincare. They give you a nice, long relaxing break, have powerful active ingredients, and manage and cure your basic problems.

SERUMS

Highly concentrated in active ingredients and quickly absorbed by your skin, they complete or enhance the action of the treatment you use on top of them. Take advantage of these products year-round as preventive medicine or as a cure for tired skin.

CREAMS

A texture star, creams are the queen of hydrating and anti-age treatments. These can be very thick and rich and are available in multiple varieties for perfect adaptation to your individual needs.

LOTIONS

More liquid than creams, these penetrate quickly into skin. They are ideal for use on your body since you can get dressed immediately after application.

FLUIDS

Thin and light, fluids, which are also called emulsions, are intended for combination skin or for very warm climates.

GELS

Most often transparent, they do not leave a greasy film on the skin and provide a cooling sensation.

OILS

Ideal for making your skin look satiny (a very sexy glossy effect), dry oils penetrate quickly without leaving behind a greasy residue.

SPRAYS

Light and fresh, these can be used in the blink of an eye. They're perfect for sunblock that you apply repeatedly and for areas that are difficult to reach, such as the back. Men love them.

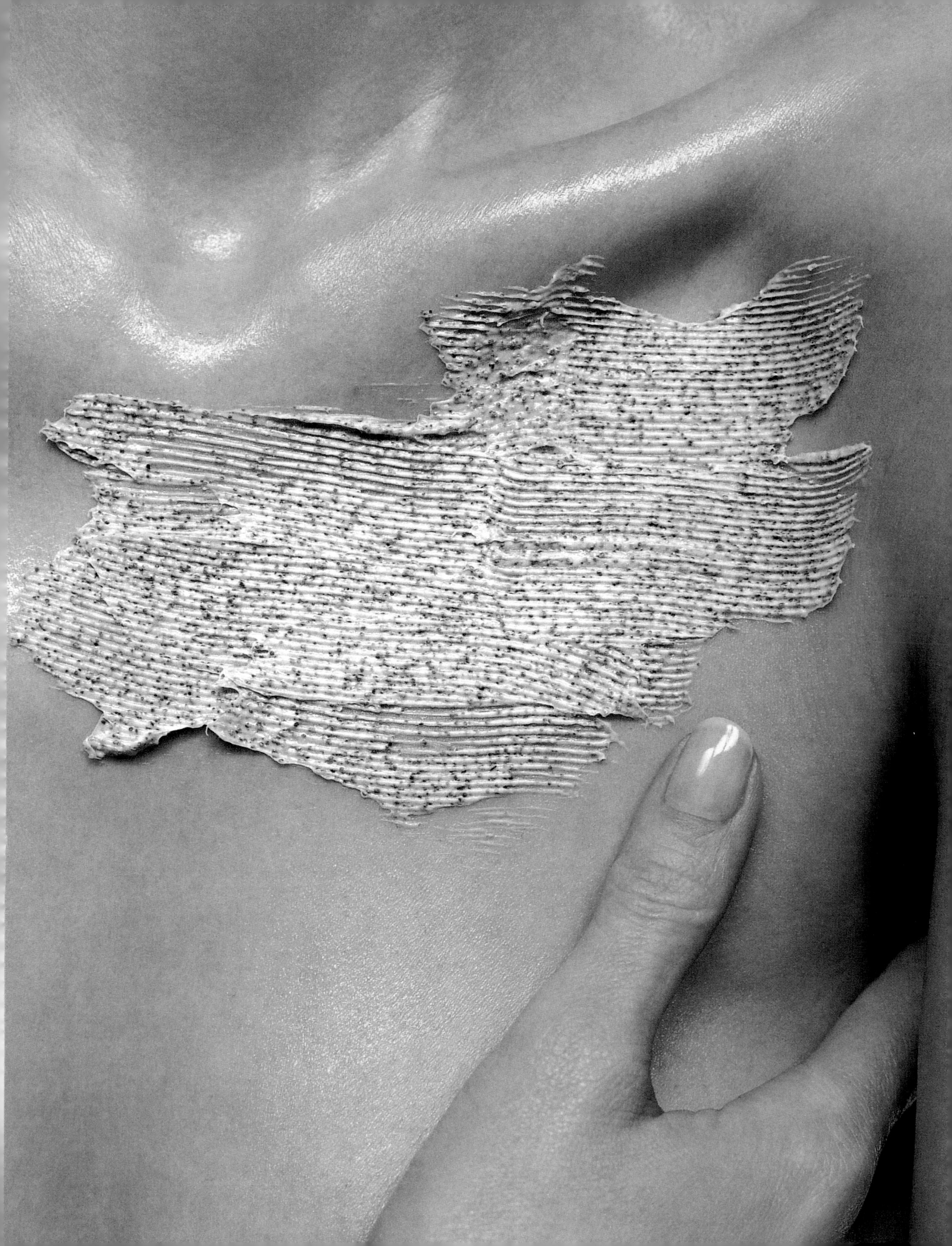

Staying on target

Is it possible to hunt down our number one hereditary enemy, cellulite? Certainly, but be reasonable and keep your feminine curves! Losing unattractive and unhealthy fat is one thing, but don't obsess over that extra pound or two!

THE GRACE OF FORMS

As luck would have it, **our body shape** and size is determined by our hormones. The fat cells in the exposed areas fill up below the waist (this is the pear-shaped type, whereas most men develop fat in the stomach area, resulting in the apple-shaped type) before moving to other parts of the body. Almost no women are spared this phenomenon, and even the thinnest among us have the right to some padding.

Depending on our metabolism, fatty tissue represents **10%–25% of our weight.** It is made up of cells with an elevated lipid content, adipocytes, which are grouped together in fatty corpuscles imprisoned in a network of connective partitions traversed by blood vessels and lymphatic vessels as well as nerve fibers. They contain 10%–15% water.

The **adipocyte** is an expandable cell capable of stocking a large quantity of fat, and its **volume can increase 27 times.** The stockpiling of fats in the adipocytes is made in the form of **triglycerides,** molecules synthesized in the adipocyte from glucose and free fatty acids. This is the principle of lipogenesis; the opposite, **lipolysis,** causes the depletion of the stockpile of fats. But under the influence of many factors (hormones, food intake that is higher than the energy demand of the organism), **lipogenesis** increases. It creates an imbalance of stocking and depleting, which is the origin of the formulation and appearance of cellulite. ▶

Do you have a bit of padding around the middle? Simply pinch your skin between two fingers at the waist; measure the pinch and divide by two to find out the thickness of the fatty layer. If you get more than a half an inch, the answer is yes!

ADVICE FROM A DOCTOR
There have been many definitions of cellulite proposed in the past by doctors. The most precise: hydrolipidostrophy, which denotes both the accumulation of fatty cells and the increase of water trapped in the tissues.

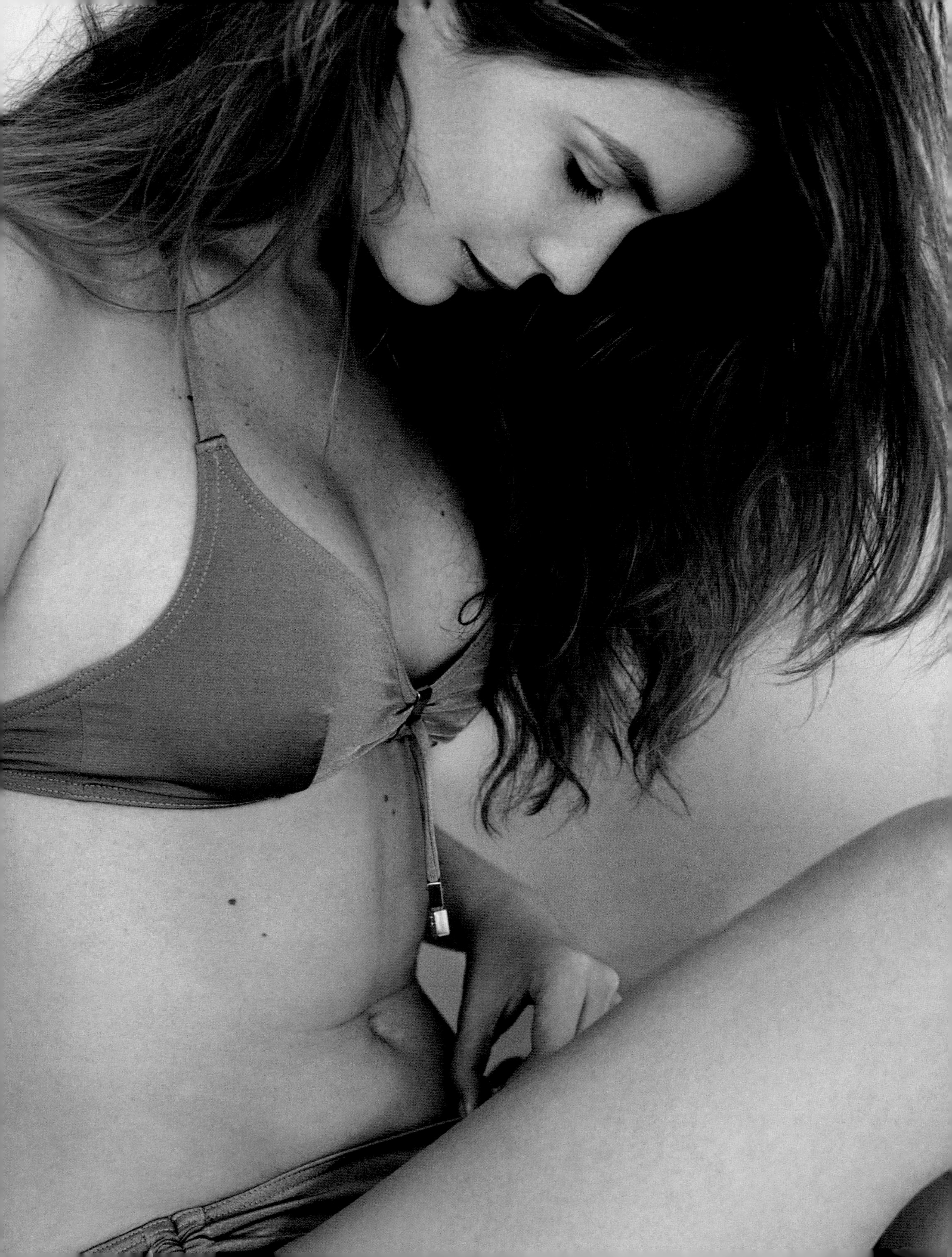

Taking matters into your own hands

Tackling problem areas head-on will yield results, as long as you don't give up. Take charge of your daily routine. The key? Targeted massage for smooth, toned skin and a genuine impact on cellulite and varicose veins.

Lower the heat; your body will use more energy if it has to fight the cold.

Water represents only 30% of the weight in our adipose tissue. Losing weight is exhausting! That's why it's so important to drink more to facilitate the work of the kidneys in eliminating impurities.

ADVICE FROM A DOCTOR
"Orange skin" is another name for superficial cellulite, the opposite of deep cellulite, which causes you to become fat. It constitutes a true padding that uniformly covers the lower extremities, the pelvis, and also the upper body. It fills with water and gets trapped in the layers of fibrous tissue, which prevent microcirculation from occurring properly. It is very sensitive to female hormones, particularly progesterone. This is what gives skin a bumpy look.

GET YOUR CELLULITE TO SURRENDER!

Every day after you shower, for a minimum of four weeks, apply a slimming cream or gel rich in active ingredients (caffeine, bitter orange, ivy, horse chestnut, ginkgo biloba, calcium, soy extract) to drain and deplete cellulite and promote the decrease in water retention and the elimination of toxins. The effects of these are **boosted by massage.**

A good starter: dietary additions that block fats and help to flush water out of your system: black currant, green tea, dandelion.

CLASSIC MASSAGE

Using a circular motion, start at your ankles, work up to your thighs, and end with your hips and buttocks.

ULTRAPRO: MANUAL VEIN DRAINAGE

This consists of chasing the water imprisoned in the tissues in your veins, reestablishing the difference in pressure that allows the blood flow to find its logical direction once more. The deep network (in the muscles) and the superficial network (between the muscles and the skin) communicate via siphons (perforans), which you stimulate with massage.

Seated, with your legs stretched out in front of you, bend back the leg to be massaged and begin at the inside of the foot, then work upward toward your groin inside the lower leg and thigh. Repeat 10 times, stretching the leg out straight when you reach the groin. **For the front of the thigh,** work up from the outer knee to the inner groin. **For the outer thigh,** start at your saddlebags and work down to the back of the knee. **For the lower leg**—calf, knee, and ankle—always work from bottom to top. And **for the hips,** work from outer to inner hips toward the groin. Finish with **your feet in the air,** lying on your back, and scissor your legs like windshield wipers.

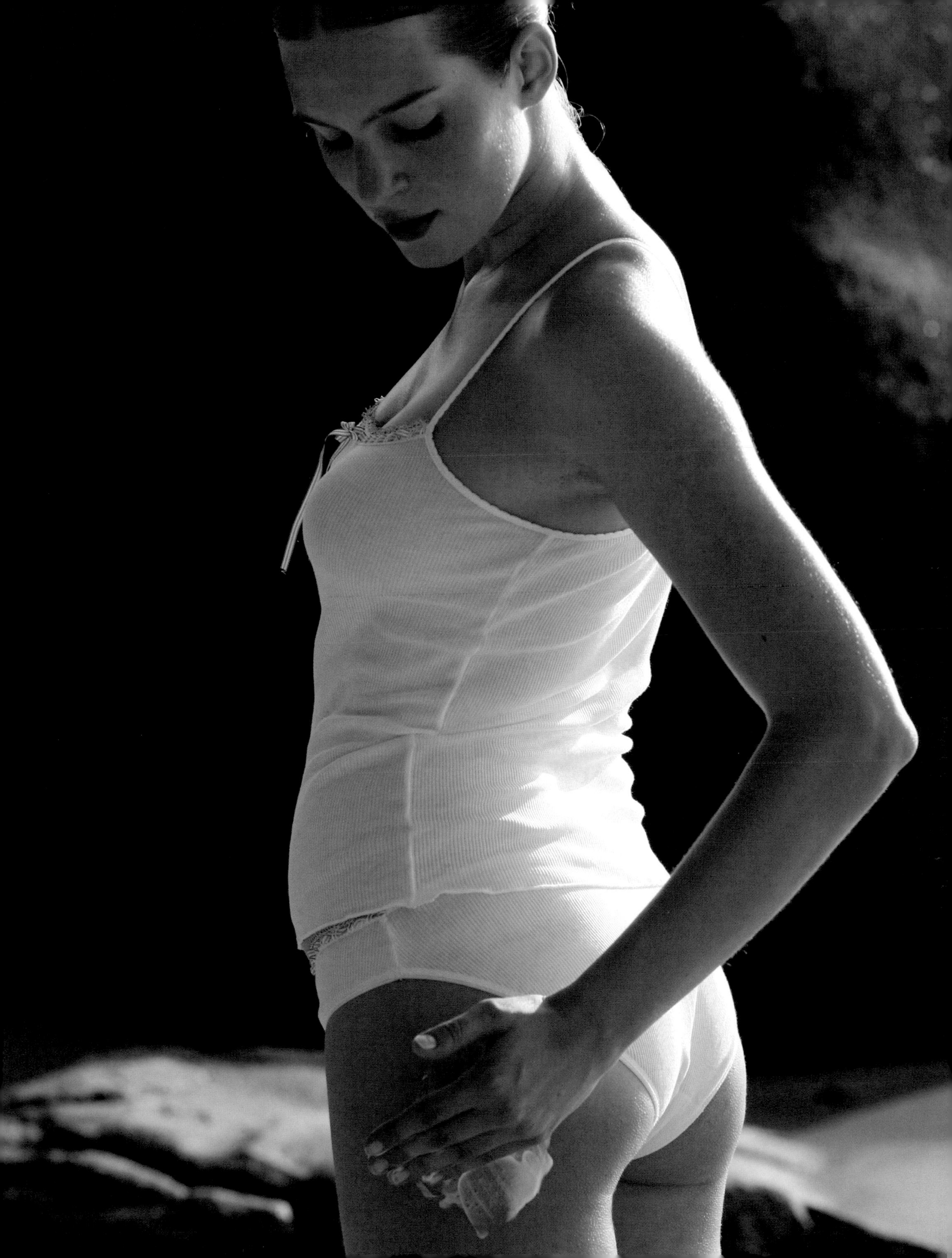

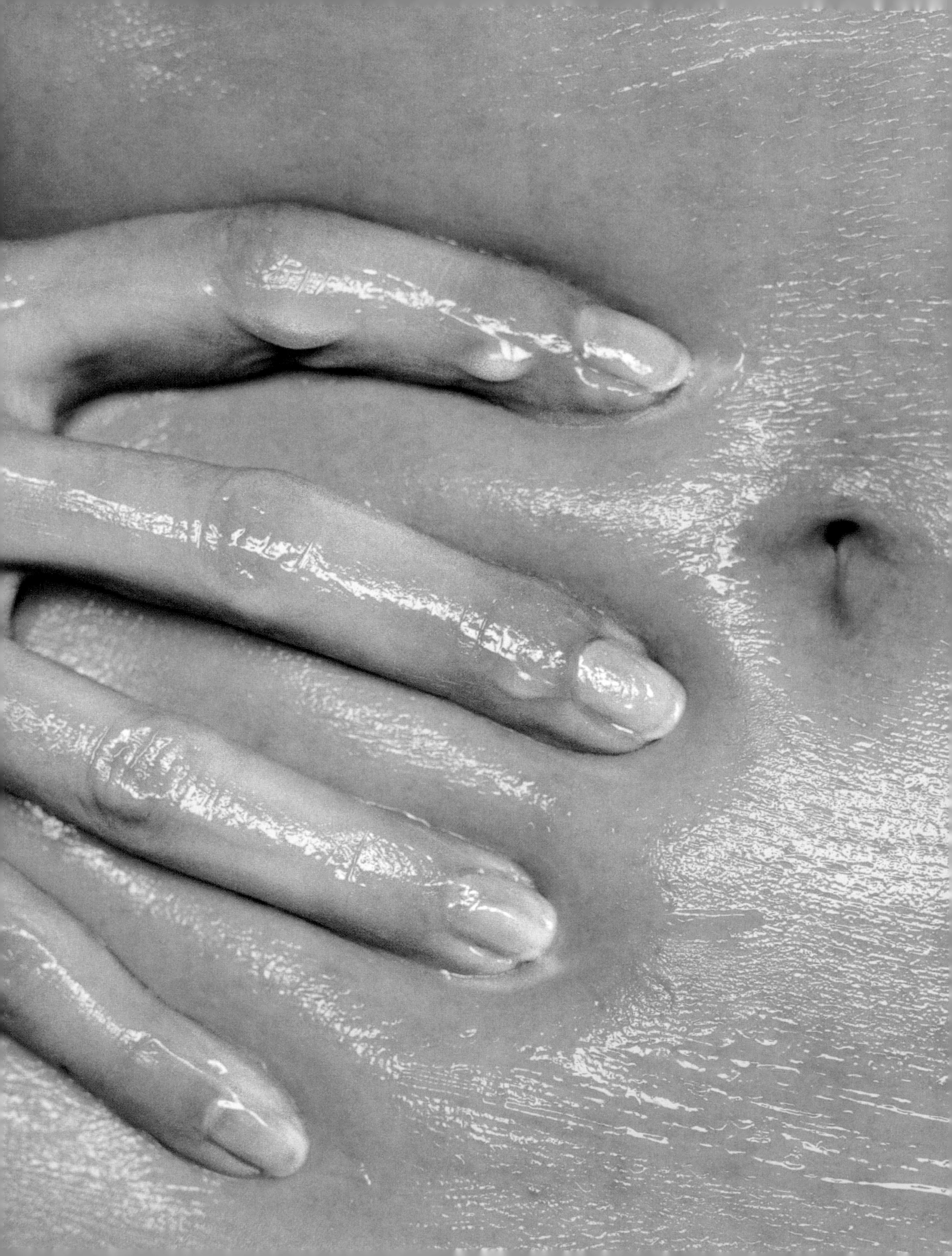

Liposuction: fact and fiction

Liposuction consists of tried and tested techniques based on a strongly esthetic but rigorously medical approach. Here's a quick list of options explained.

Begin by correcting everything that can aggravate your case (**hormonal imbalances** and **circulation problems**).

Injections, ultrasounds, massage, lymphatic drainage Aside from going to the gym and playing sports, try some other treatments that destroy the sclerotic barrier. **Mesotherapy** (an injection of products with a very short needle) works well on localized cellulite.

The stomach, the spot where reserves of fat love to make their home, is also an area that undergoes a great deal of tension, and distension, mainly from pregnancies, which stretch the skin and the muscular casings. An ultrasound scan will clearly evaluate the state of these places.

What to do? If you have a little tummy, **liposuction,** using a local anesthetic, will effectively resolve the problem, but we all know that surgery is always serious and will sometimes only be an option for people with larger amounts of fat. **Lipolaser,** or **laser lipolysis,** is the ultimate perfection of years of research, and its benefits are now recognized by all. It can be done on an outpatient basis without any follow-up visits, and the patient can return to work the next day.

When there are several problems (stomach wall and skin distended, with a thick layer of fat as a result), **abdominal plastic surgery** is required. The fat is removed, usually by **liposuction,** the muscles are tightened if needed, and the excess skin is cut away. This is a serious intervention and is not without risks—and it leaves quite a scar. Think twice before signing up for this!

ADVICE FROM A SURGEON

WHEN THE MUSCULAR CASING HAS BECOME LOOSE: This is seen in the middle of the abdomen as an enlargement of the area where the right and left muscles are joined (diastasis recti) that supports the front of the chest since there is almost no fat to lose or remove. The solution consists of tightening this central area of the abdomen with the help of an incision that will be hidden under a bathing suit. When the fat is on the interior of the abdomen (featuring a prominent stomach and more than a 30 inch waist), you are facing a metabolic syndrome generally associated with problems of high quantities of sugar and fats in the blood, as well as hypertension. This is a medical problem that needs to be addressed.

The buttocks This area is the most complex and so the most intriguing to doctors. All the difficulty of treatment comes from the fact that the muscles are "suspended" on a fixed frame and must bear their own weight.

A pouch at your knee? A notorious area for stockpiling fat, your knees are at the mercy of your hormones. An inflammation can promote the transformation of certain cells into adipocytes, stimulating lipogenesis (puffiness at these reservoirs through the production of fat).

ADVICE FROM A DOCTOR Before any intervention, an extensive consultation, as with any procedure done under anesthesia, is highly recommended.

▶ TEXTBOOK CASE: THE BUTTOCKS

Gaining weight means stretching the envelope holding the extra pounds. Pay attention to **buttock ptosis** (sagging bottom), which can make you look heavier. Improve the appearance of this area by using sculpting exercises: the muscles in this area can be strengthened by using a table inclined 35 to 45 degrees to counter your weight, and by contracting the affected muscles (the gluteals). You can also try a variety of techniques: **lipolysis** or **lipolaser** will help to reduce the volume, **lipofilling** will add volume to an area, and **lipolaser** will retighten the area. **Liposuction** under general anesthesia is also an option, but the benefits must be weighed against the risks.

LEG WORK: STRESS-FREE LIPO

Liposculpture is another ambulatory procedure that associates the effectiveness of liposuction (elimination of fat by sucking) with the gentleness of a procedure performed under local anesthesia in a surgical setting but without the need to miss work. **Lipolaser** is best for deep or extensive cellulite. Less serious an ordeal than liposuction, it is now growing in popularity. **Lipolysis** may be proposed for small amounts of localized cellulite (saddlebags, knees) and works well on "orange skin" (there is no sucking of fat involved) associated with endermology since it helps to smooth the surface of the skin.

Classic liposuction is not a method to lose weight but rather a method to lose inches in abnormally or disproportionately developed areas. Liposculpture is done using a cannula connected to a vacuum. At the end of a session (which lasts 2.5 hours maximum), support hose or support panties must be worn for at least three weeks. The inner thighs are the most delicate to treat; you must be very attentive to the quality of the skin.

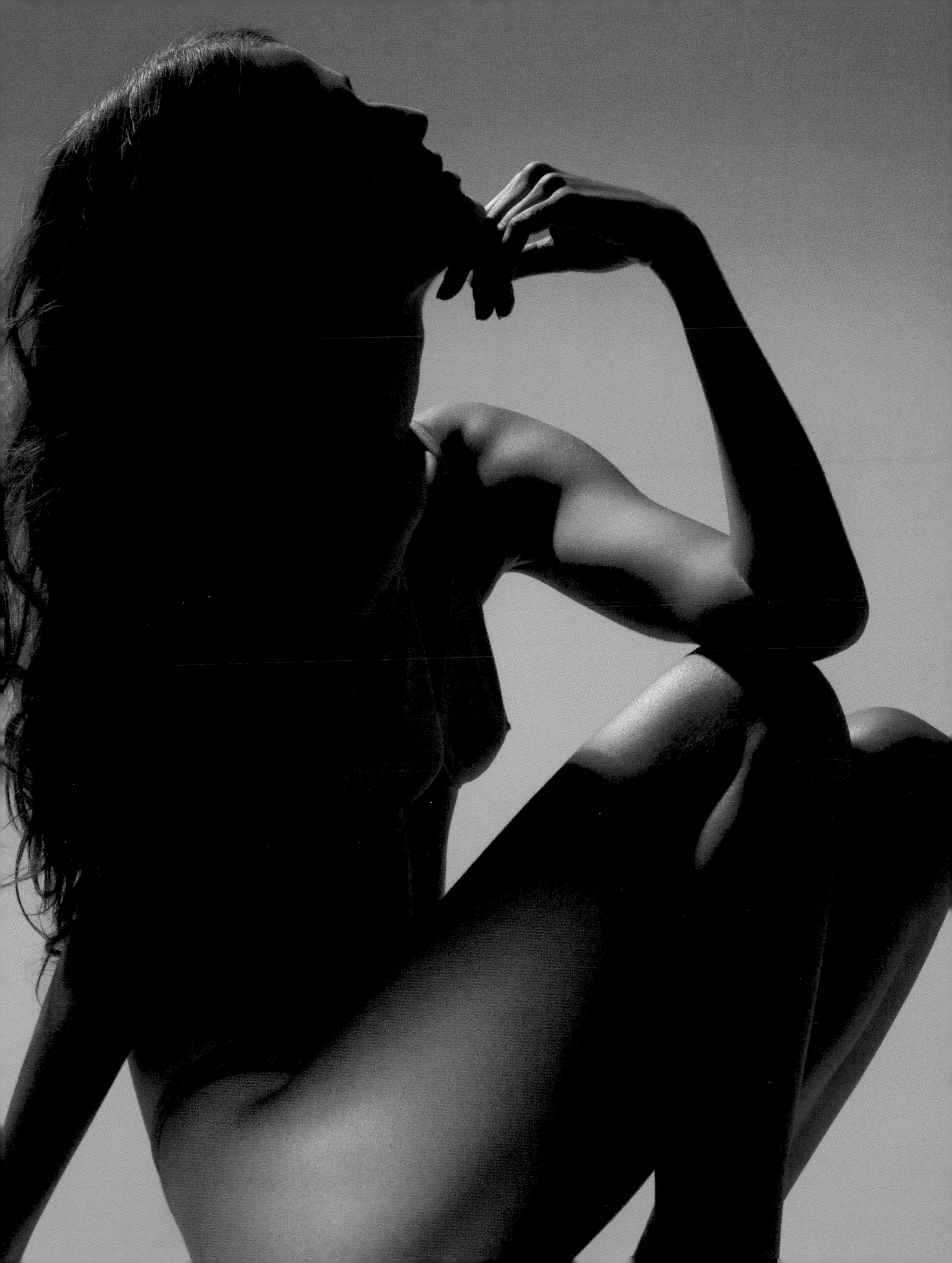

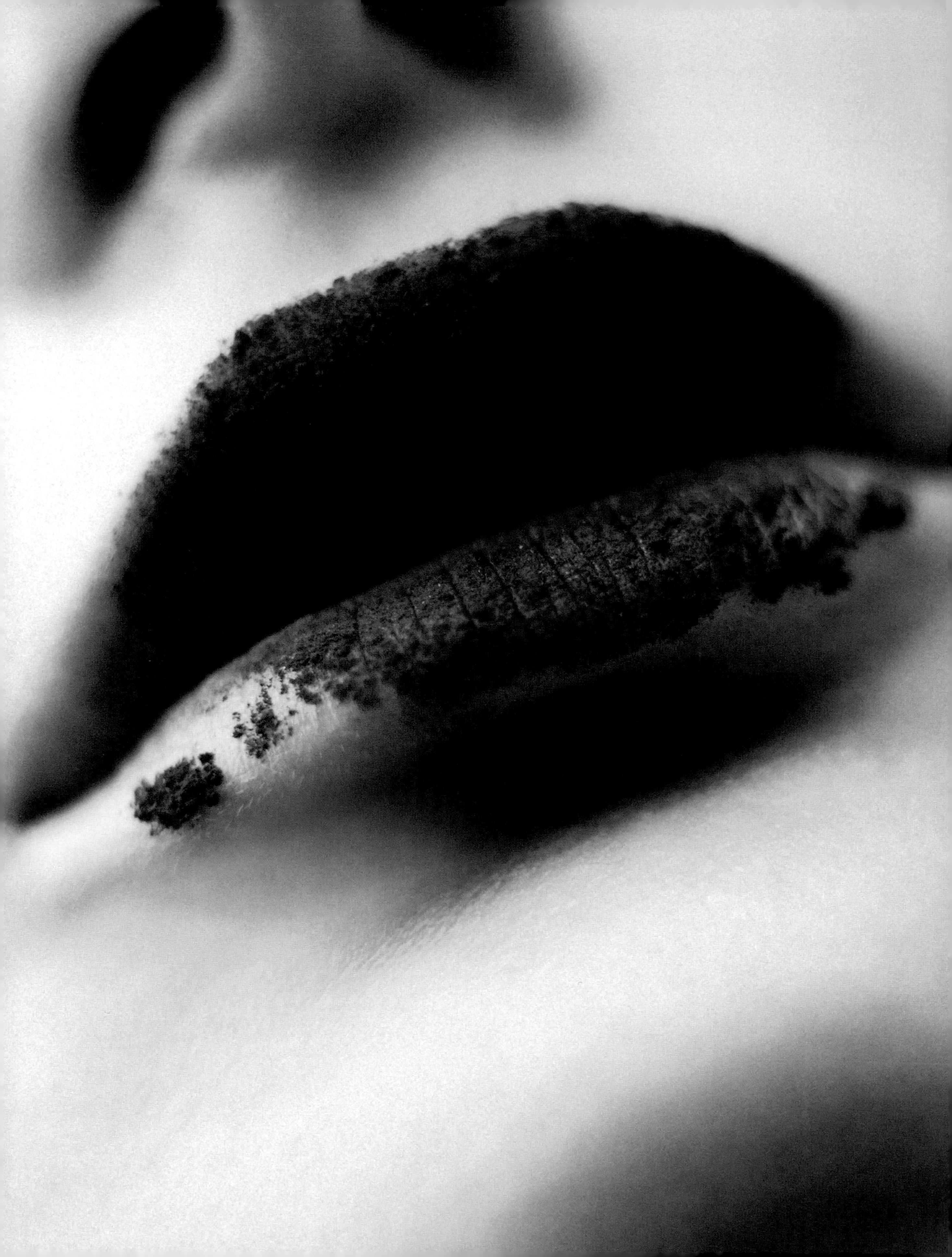

Take a bite out of life by enjoying healthy foods

Eat to your Health

A healthy, well-balanced diet is the basis for everything. It allows you to fuel your body beautifully.

Slim down where I want?
This is the objective of morphonutrition:
- Too much sugar will develop breasts and thighs.
- Too much starchy foods and carbohydrates will develop the stomach.
- Too much protein will develop the chest and muscles.

Lose weight? Maybe later!
The principle of chrononutrition rests on finding a dietary rhythm based on demand. Eat good fats in the morning accompanied by proteins packing a kick-starting punch, a full lunch, a light afternoon snack, and a very light evening meal.

ADVICE FROM A DIETICIAN

THE BEST SPICES
Cinnamon helps lower the level of sugar in the blood. Ginger warms the senses with more than 40 antioxidant compounds. It also assists in the digestion of garlic and onion when eaten in the same meal, for an optimal effect of beneficial nutrients. Turmeric is also excellent (see page 117).

DON'T DEPRIVE YOURSELF!

You'll get indigestion from fad diets or starving yourself. Today, the top priority is to choose the best foods to nourish your beautiful machine, which will have the greatest benefit for its motor: your brain. A clear mind comes from a healthy body that works longer and better when properly nourished.

The key is **not to eat less, but to eat better.** Choose foods that are rich in protective substances—fiber, antioxidants, magnesium, vitamins and minerals, phytoestrogens, and healthy fats (omega–3s). A healthy diet takes care of your intestines, which are your second "brain" and alert you to the first signs of a problem. Your intestines provide the means to absorb the benefits all these healthy treats.

PRO PROBIOTICS?

Probiotics are living microorganisms that, when administered in adequate quantities, produce a beneficial effect on the health of the host organism—you! The intestines have many functions for digestion, absorption, defense, and tolerance. An imbalance in the bacterial flora present in the large and small intestine due to stress, poor diet, or medication causes immediate discomfort as well as more long-term health risks. Probiotics restore the bacterial flora, improve the workings of the intestines, and allow better absorption of nutrients.

TELL ME WHAT YOU ATE...

Our **morphology** is in part due to our diet. All this is tempered by the role of hormonal receptors located in the adipocytes, as well as heredity and ethnicity. ▶

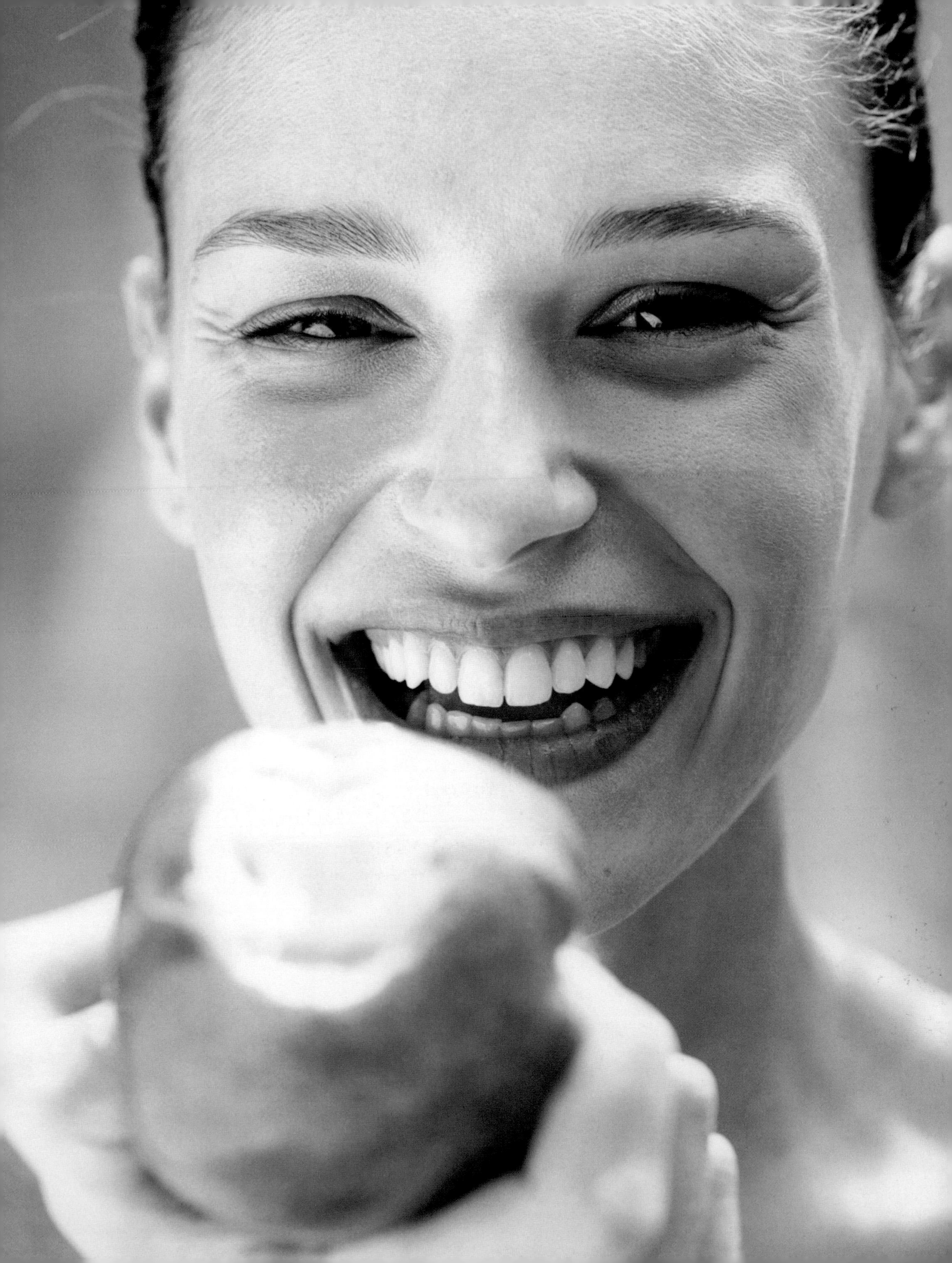

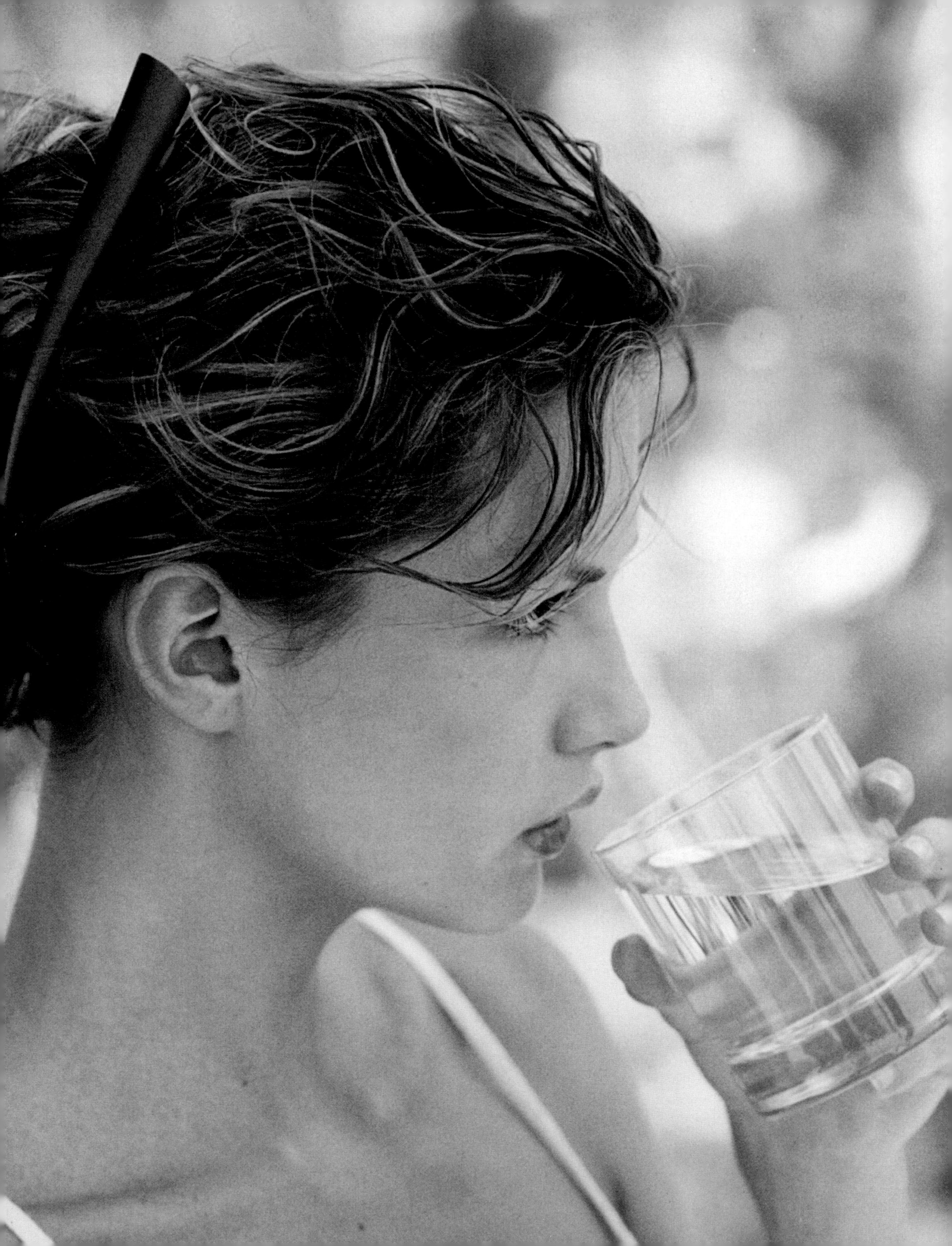

▶ OKINAWA: LONGEVITY IS ON THE MENU

The Okinawan diet provides all the benefits of Japanese cuisine—only better, including more variety and less salt. For the past 30 years, we have been studying the way of life and diet of the inhabitants of this archipelago, situated on the spice route, off the coast of Japan. Renowned for their longevity and proverbial health, they eat small meals composed of many vegetables, oily fish, soy products, seaweeds, brown rice, sweet potatoes, no dairy or wheat products (and therefore no glutens), no sugar, and very little salt. Moreover, they have excellent stress management (see tai chi on page 160).

Unknown to the Japanese, the spice turmeric, a cousin of ginger, is widely used there. Turmeric is a "multi-anti"—anti-inflammatory, antimicrobial, antiviral, anti-infection, antitumor, and antiparasitic.

Cretan diets, which are similar to Okinawan ones, add red wine (in moderation, for the benefits of **resveratrol**) and olive oil (which has flavonoid **antioxidants**).

ALL ABOUT OMEGAS

More than 60% of our brain is made up of lipids, of which more than 70% are omega-3s, since the fats are formed by different fatty acids. A good balance between them is critical to maintain good health. Keep saturated fats to a minimum, and consume **five times more omega-6 than omega-3.**

Saturated fatty acids: fatty meats, cold cuts, sweets, and cheese.

Monounsaturated fatty acids: olive oil.

Omega-3 polyunsaturated fatty acids: grapeseed oil, oily fish.

Omega-6 polyunsaturated fatty acids: sunflower oil (but omega-6s are also prevalent in packaged foods, margarine, and cookies).

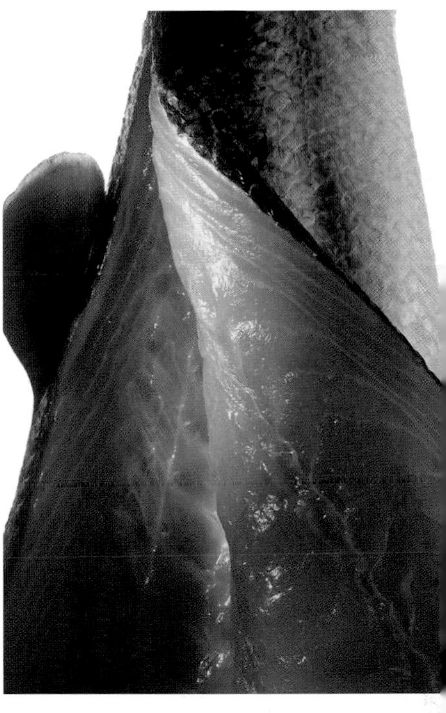

ADVICE FROM A DIETICIAN

KEY POINTS

Drink 50 ounces of water enriched with calcium and magnesium per day. Don't deprive yourself of starchy foods; it's a terrible mistake. These are critical suppliers of energy via complex carbohydrates, and you should eat them in appropriate amounts.

Fiber, vitamins, and anti-aging delights

Making time for healthy habits is as good for the morale as it is for glowing skin, beautiful hair, strong nails, and a shapely figure.

MAKING A DAILY APPEARANCE AT YOUR TABLE . . .

• Fruits and vegetables in a variety of soups, salads, gratins, and compotes.

• A small green salad at one of your meals dressed with healthy oils (60% olive and 40% grapeseed oil, organic and cold-pressed).

• Proteins—meat, fish, eggs—in the morning or afternoon. You should eat oily fish two or three times a week.

• Nuts and dried fruits—figs, prunes, apricots. These go well in salads.

• Green tea, rich in polyphenols.

• A light meal in the evening, but one that contains complex carbohydrates.

• A glass and a half of good red wine every day. If you drink coffee, go easy on it and buy organic—pesticides become concentrated in your cup.

ANTIOXIDANTS: A BANQUET OF COLORS

The **reds, yellows,** and **oranges** (peppers, apples, tomatoes, citrus fruits, peaches, carrots) offer **carotenoids, lycopene,** and **lutein.**

The **purples** and **violets** (red cabbage, beets, figs, prunes, raisins, raspberries, currants) offer **anthocyanins.**

The **greens** (salad greens, spinach, cabbage) offer **chlorophyll;** the green may be hidden by warmer colors, but it's there, along with its benefits.

CHOCOLATE: GUILTY PLEASURE?

Some of its molecules can lead to addiction . . . but we're definitely hooked on the joy of eating it!

ADVICE FROM A DIETICIAN

Dried oily nuts that are not roasted or salted (walnuts, hazelnuts, almonds, cashews, macadamias, and pistachios) are rich in healthy fats, calcium, and magnesium and, when eaten in reasonable quantities, will not cause you to gain weight. In fact, their fiber and mineral salts actually prevent some fat absorption.

Frozen vegetables? Half of the vitamins in fresh vegetables evaporate after two days on display in the grocery store. But that doesn't mean you have to go to the market every day to benefit from what veggies have to offer. You can reap the rewards of vegetables from the freezer case, which are just waiting to be defrosted!

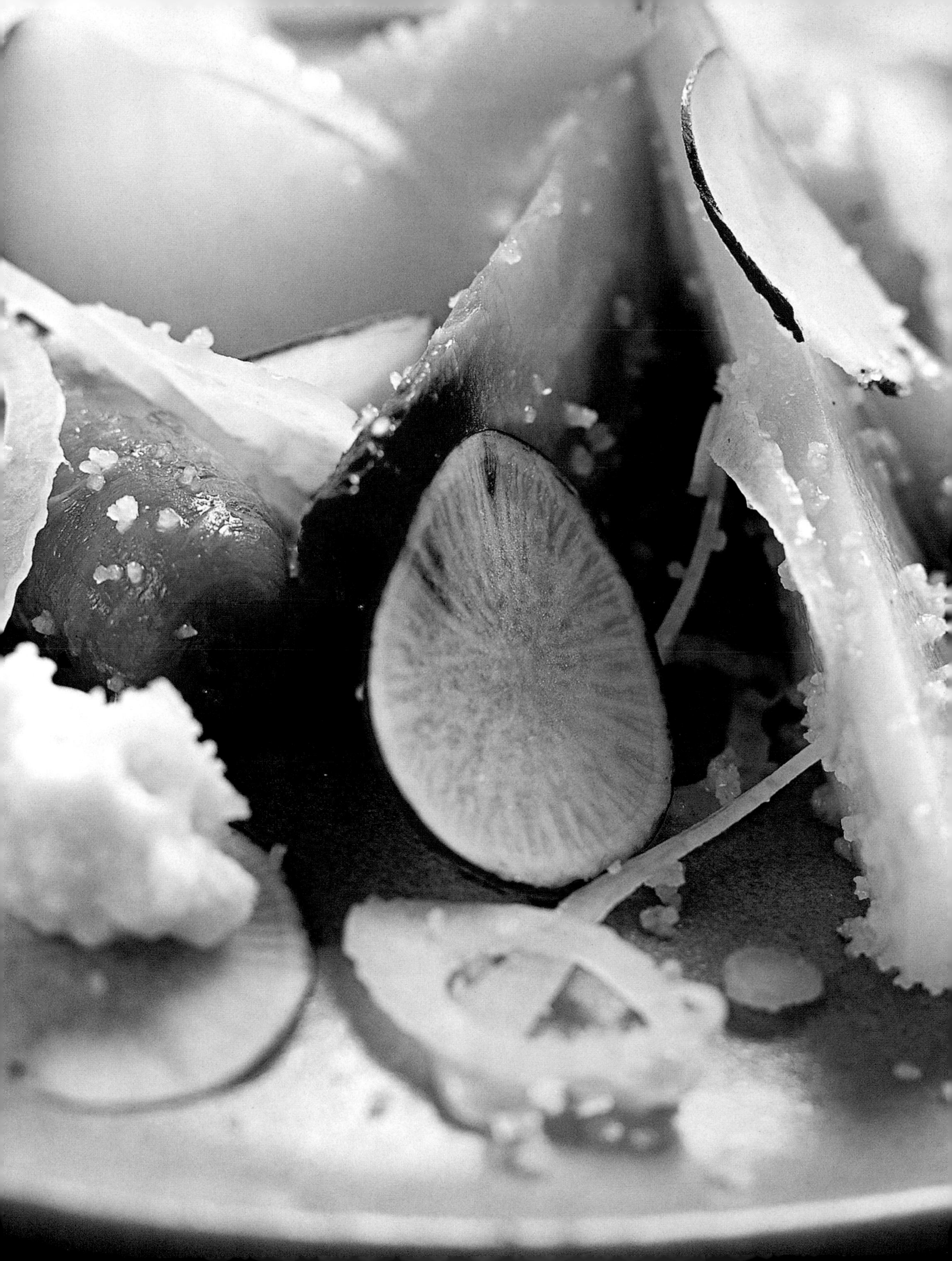

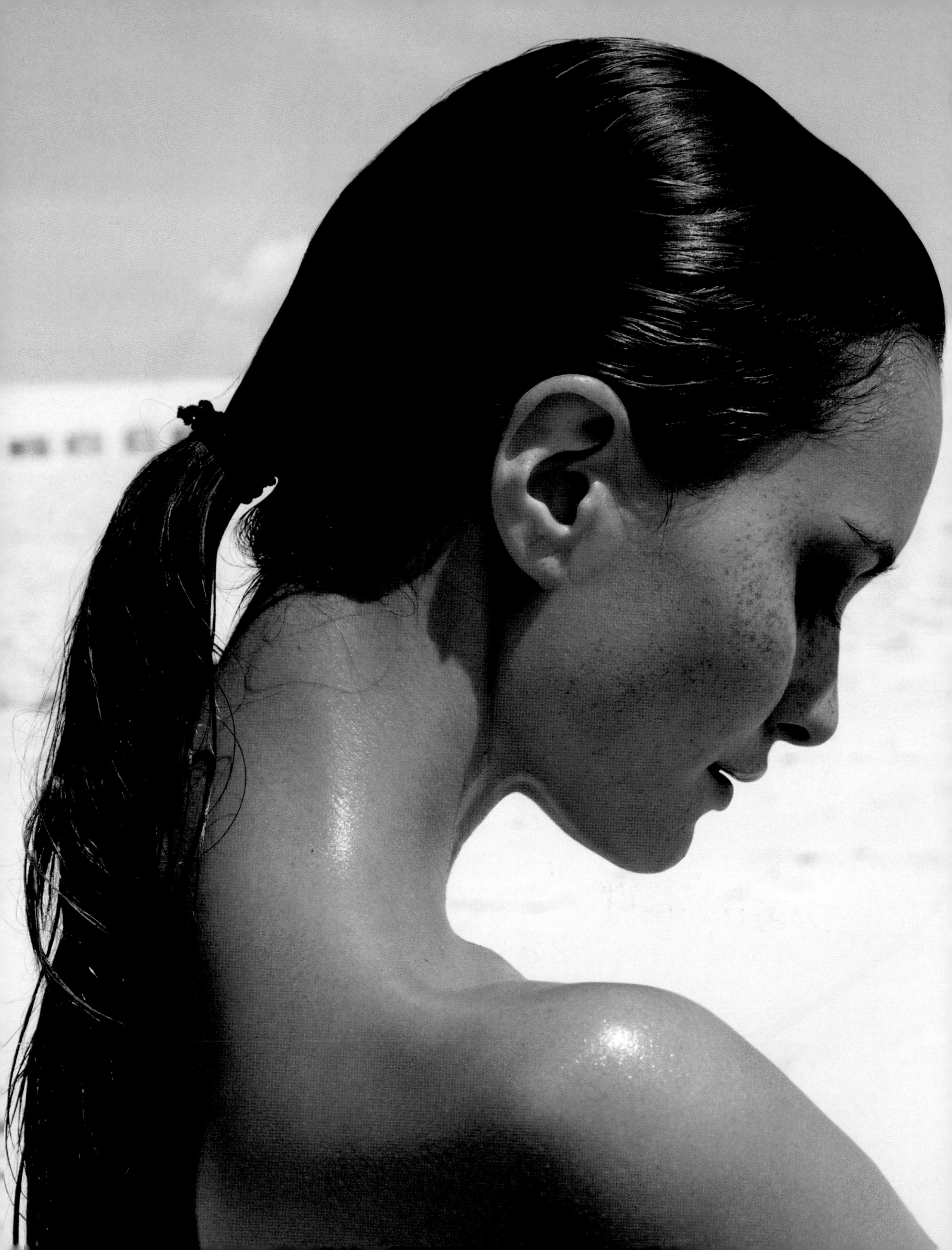

Work with and conspire against age

How old is your skin?

The first of its kind, the biological skin laboratory directed by Professor Philippe Humbert, Chief of Dermatology at the Saint-Jacques Hospital in Besançon, France, offers a personalized approach to aging gracefully.

Is an exam of your skin's surface and structure more precise than a medical exam? One can calculate the relief of the skin and evaluate its "mechanical" properties (based on genetics and age). Sags and jowls appear on one person; wrinkles or bags under the eyes on another. If you use collagen, will it reactivate your microcirculation or stimulate your production of elastin?

Thanks to instruments that analyze the skin's image, doctors can characterize the type of aging and plan the best therapeutic approach, including the choice of cosmetics, to respond precisely to each individual case. They cannot prescribe the same method or advise the use of the same active ingredient to every woman over 45.

The **elasticity of the skin** is reduced with age while its **expandability** increases (about 5% every 10 years).

Relief: This measurement allows a doctor to assess the roughness of skin and count the furrows and plateaus of the surface.

Tone and brightness: These are measured with an optical device that studies the reflection of light on the skin.

Microcirculation: This is quantified by the analysis of the small skin vessels seen using video skin scoping. A tiny camera observes the capillary vessels using transillumination. Their number and distribution **depend partly on the shade of the skin and its tone.**

Level of hydration: An electrical measurement called capacitance classifies dry skin according to an index (a level of hydration less than 40 means very dry skin).

Level of sebum secretion: A sebumeter uses a method based on image analysis. ▶

Aesthetic dermatology, recognized by the French Association of Dermatologists, is practiced by doctors who undergo rigorous and scientific training. The treatments offered are very effective. It is critical that a precise exam is first completed to determine and define the type of aging; later, the effects of the treatments used are closely monitored. Little by little, dermatology offices are becoming better equipped with diagnostic tools that use bioengineering methods, biometrics, and quantitative imagery.

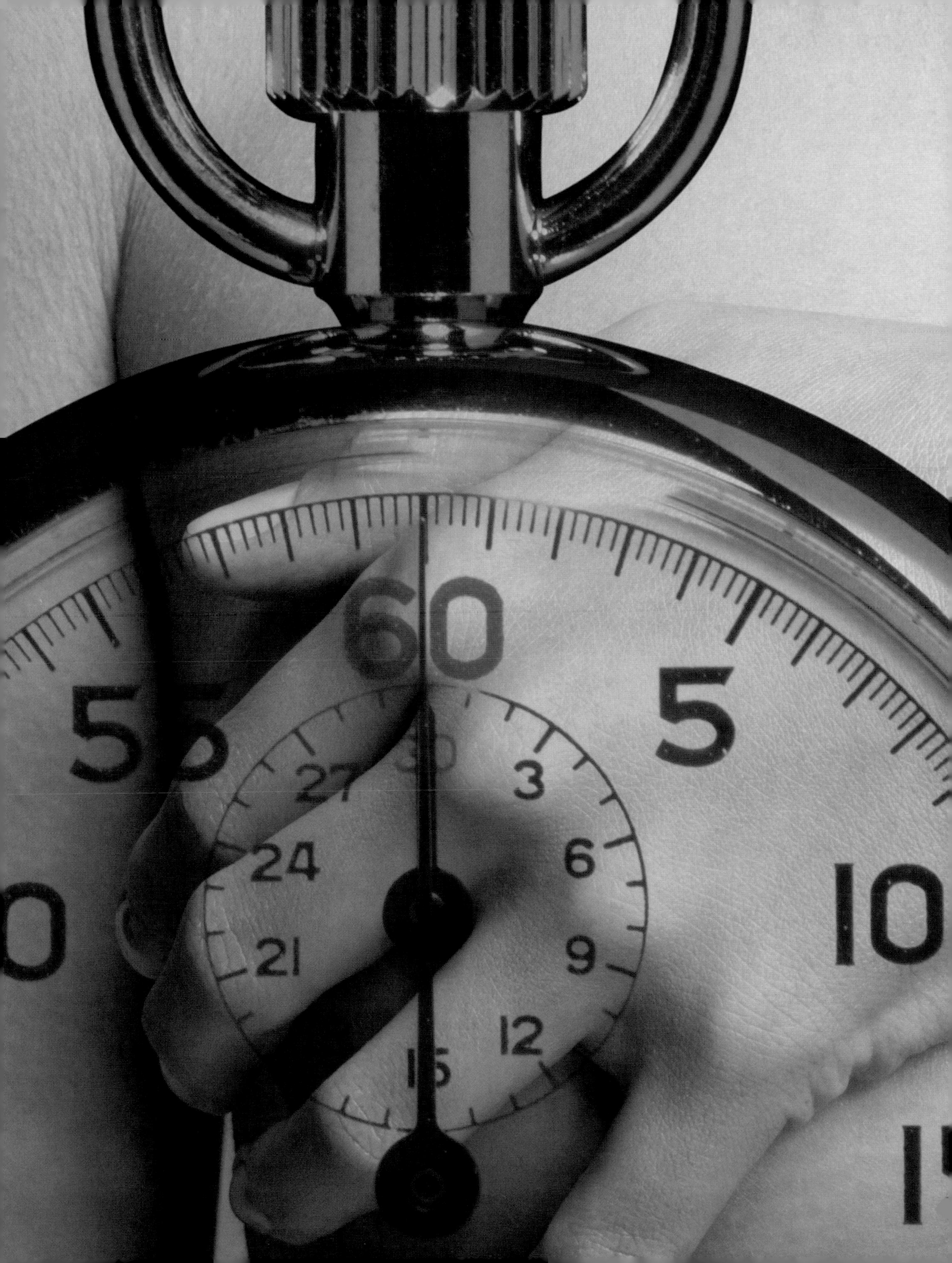
55
60
5
10
30
3
6
9
12
15
21
24
27

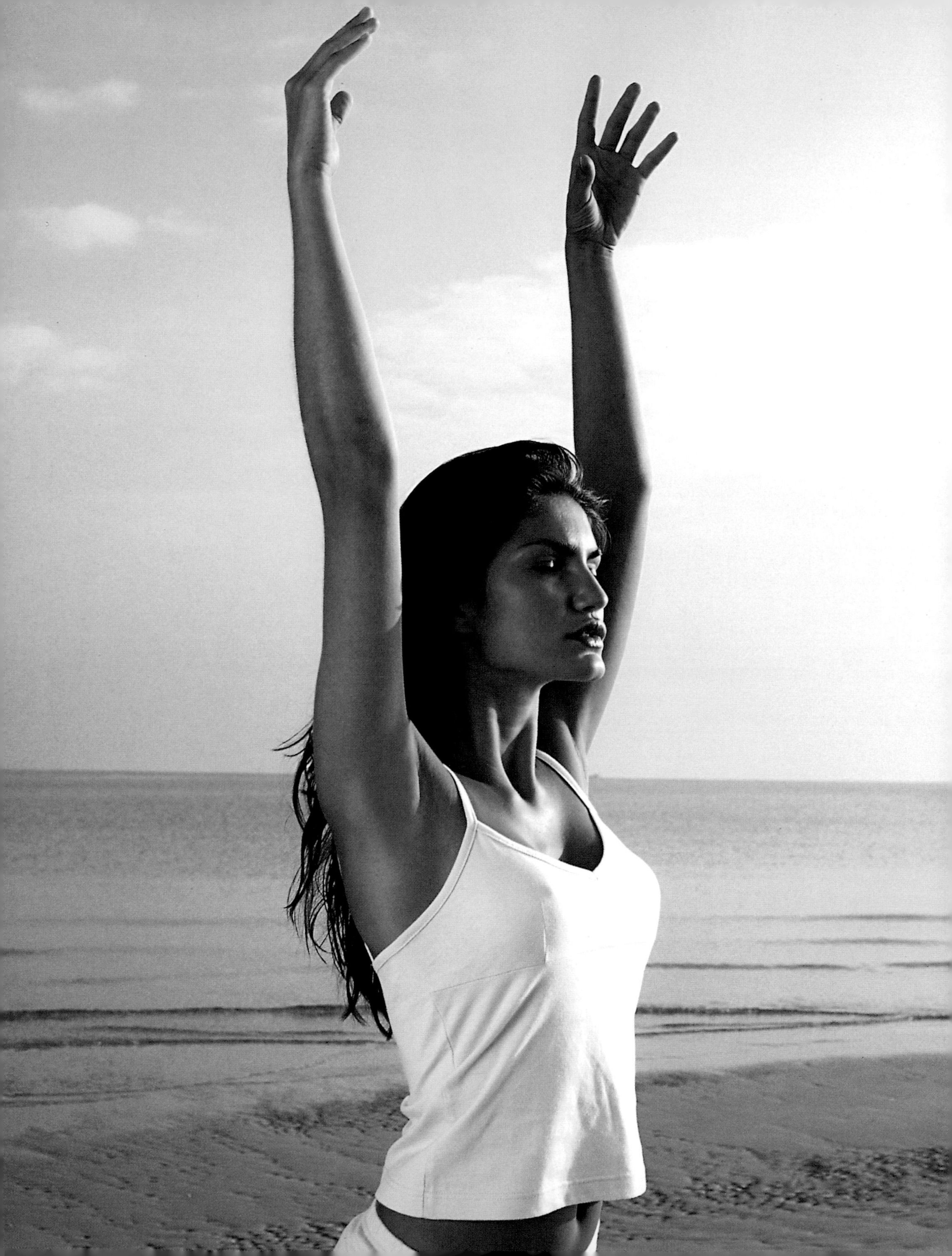

▶ THE GOLDEN RULES FOR PREVENTING THE ATTACKS OF TIME

Controlling aging is first and foremost a matter of protection and prevention. Sun protection, quitting smoking, and eliminating stress all contribute to the health of your skin. Hydrate it with creams, massage it, and use cosmetics that have a proven effectiveness.

You must make it a priority to care for your entire body to reestablish the equilibrium of all its functions (homeostasis)—in which balanced nutrition plays an integral role.

You must act simultaneously on every aspect of your health. Otherwise, it's like inflating one car tire and leaving the other three flat!

Cosmetology is the foundation of skin care, performing simple functions like creating a barrier or hydrating the skin. It does these thanks to special active ingredients in cosmetics working on different cellular functions that permit the reactivation of cells such as fibroblasts, where the synthesis of collagen is increased. Their action only happens with proper use over a sufficient period of time, and you must know how to combine the active ingredients for their fullest effect.

There is a **trend toward using cellular therapy as a means of taking charge of aging.** There are already cases where adipose tissue (subcutaneous fatty tissue) was removed from a patient to reinject it elsewhere to add volume. We are moving more toward cellular therapy using fibroblasts, cells that fabricate collagen in the dermis.

Stem cells, because of their great potential, have been the focus of studies in many different areas, including skin aging. However, these new methods remain difficult to make available to patients because they are expensive and still relatively experimental.

Vitamin C is essential to the maintenance of the structure of collagen. We've observed in the skin biology laboratory the decrease in the vitamin C level in skin as a function of age. The findings reveal that at age 80, the level of vitamin C in skin is decreased by 50% as compared to the skin of a 40-year-old.

A biomarker of oxidative stress, isoprostane, allows early detection to prevent maladies such as Alzheimers.

The flower of age: gathering your fruits

While we didn't learn how to extract them until the 19th century, we have known about the wonderful properties of plants since antiquity. Here's some of the latest in nutrition research.

RESVERATROL 20 IN WINE!

One of the explanations for the **French paradox** is the beneficial role played by red wine in moderate doses. We defend the richness of red wine with the benefits of **resveratrol**, a phenolic derivative present in plants that works as an antioxidant, an anticoagulant for plaque, and an anti-inflammatory; dilates veins; and prevents cellular proliferation. It gives you rosy cheeks when consumed in moderation and prolongs the life of yeast by 70%. A researcher at the University of Quebec, Frédéric Le Cren, flag waver for the antioxidant revolution, recommends it daily, whether in the form of a supplement, a bunch of grapes, or 16 ounces of grape juice. Of course, you can also drink a glass and a half of red wine! Cheers!

To fight skin's aging, the only molecule that has truly proved effective on humans, based on scientific research, is vitamin A acid (tretinoin). There are numerous cosmetic products that claim to have antioxidant properties, and in vitro studies in the lab have produced real effects that are very interesting (stimulation of collagen, slowing of the decline of elastin fibers). But the impact on human beings is more difficult to prove. The active extracts of plants such as green tea present many possibilities, but there is not enough data yet with regard to the aging of human skin.

GREEN TEA, NO TUMMY

Whether washing down sushi or to getting the morning off to the right start, you don't have to watch how much green tea you drink. It's a warrior in the battle against the accumulation of fat in the abdomen, which is as unattractive as it is unhealthy (it accelerates aging and contributes to diabetes).

POMEGRANATE: ANTIOXIDANT BOMB!

Pomegranate juice, containing a powerful antioxidant, may have the ability to fight off certain cancers, including breast cancer.

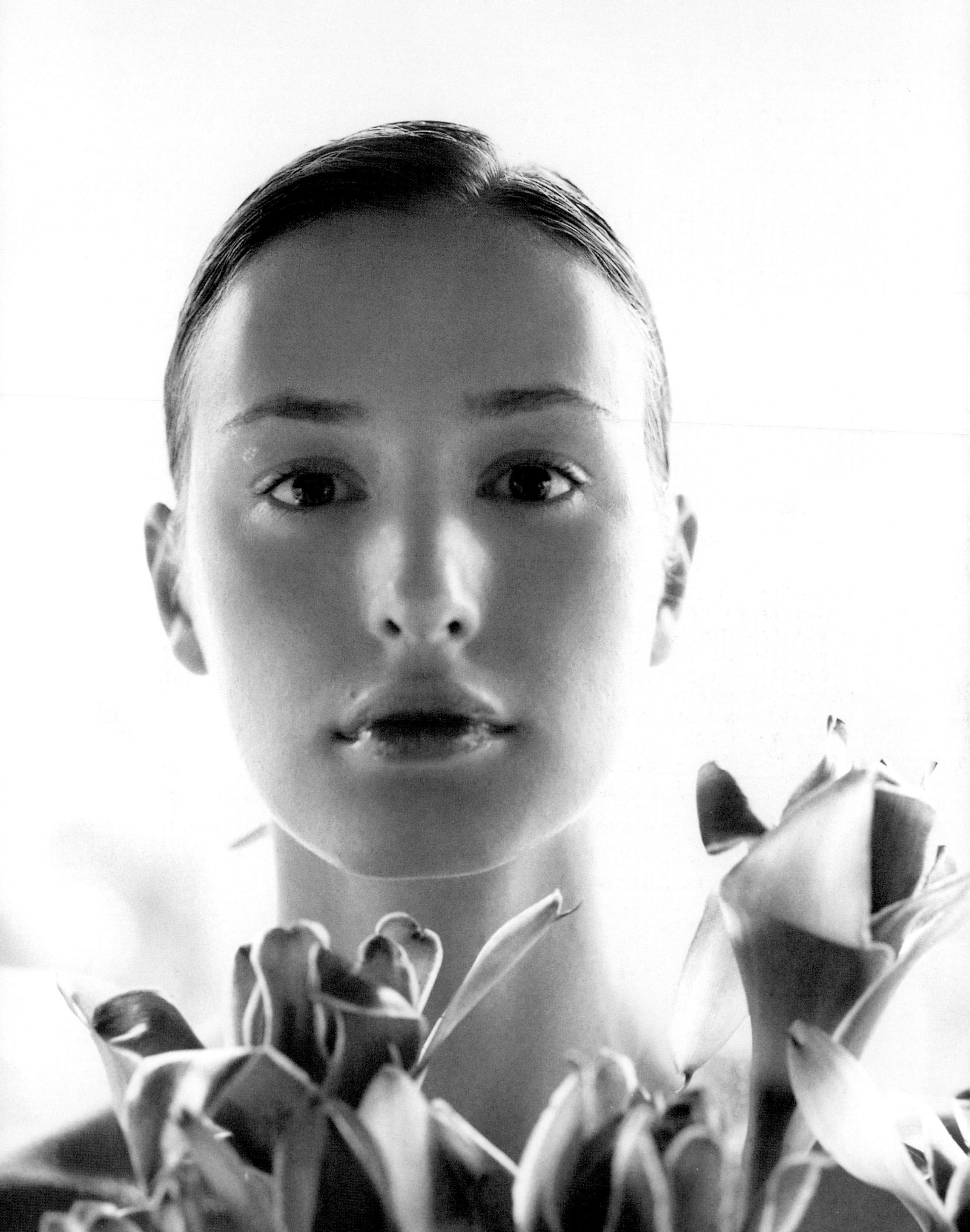

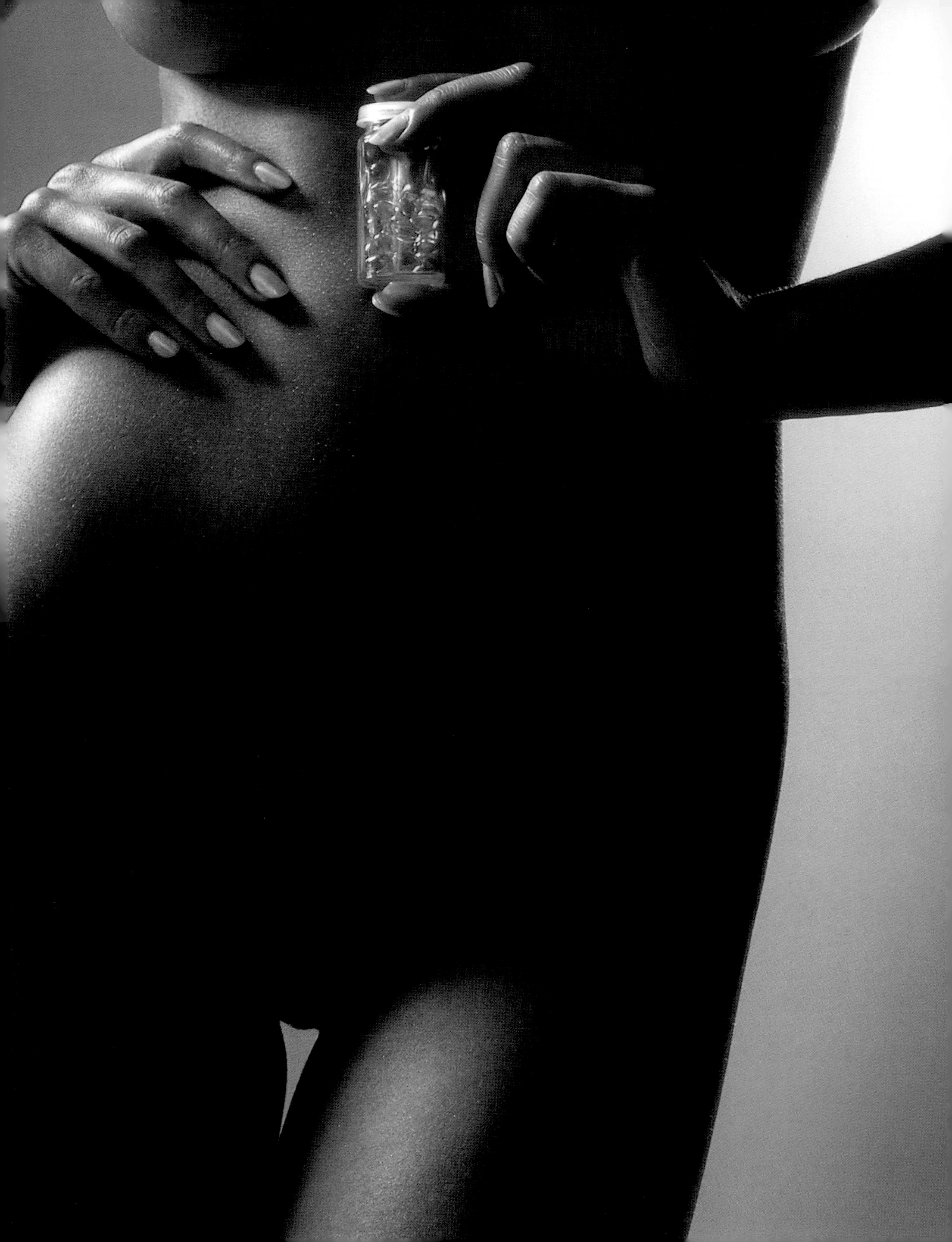

Supplements

Supplements have become more and more popular for recharging our batteries when we're dieting or to complement our food intake. The stars of this genre are, first and foremost, the vitamins and minerals found naturally in food—not the pill form!

An antioxidant medication is currently being studied to better understand the absorption of dietary supplements, and it has already proved itself in animals. As we wait, here's a glimpse of what's coming down the road.

"AMINO ACIDS FOR LIFE"—VITAMINS C AND E

Vitamin C We are unable to synthesize it, and therefore it is indispensable in the battle against infections and degenerative illnesses. Find it in citrus fruits, currant, parsley, acerola, kiwi, peppers, cauliflower, and red cabbage.

Vitamin E It slows down cellular aging and is found in wheat germ oil, soy, peanuts, olives, grains, oily fish, almonds, and hazelnuts. A single molecule of vitamin E inhibits the oxidation of 1,000 molecules of polyunsaturated fatty acids, proving it to be a very hard worker.

ANTI-AGE DREAM TEAM: SELENIUM AND ZINC

Selenium This enzyme plays a role in the stabilization of the keratin molecules in the skin and protects against the toxicity of UVA rays. Its effectiveness is increased when it is combined with vitamin E. You can get selenium from oysters, eggs, mushrooms, chicken, and carrots.

Zinc plays a role in the synthesis of collagen (as does manganese) and elastin. It stimulates the immune system and improves certain skin conditions such as psoriasis and acne. Find zinc in oysters, meats, whole grains, lentils, oily fish, walnuts, and hazelnuts.

•**Choose natural ingredients** (read the label); synthetic ingredients are less well absorbed.

•**Attention: iron and copper,** notorious oxidants, should only be used as recommended by your doctor.

Antioxidants can be beneficial as long as they are taken carefully. Research recommends a complex of many antioxidants that have complementary efficacy—taken only for a short duration. A cure over a short period of time (three weeks) before sun exposure has great advantages. However, it's not recommended to take them for months on end, especially when you're eating a good, balanced diet. Some women take them regularly—for good muscle tone, a flat stomach, or beautiful legs. These are frequently the same antioxidant molecules found in all the specialized vitamins. It is important to know that if you have too much, you can become pro-oxidative and create problems as a result.

Anti-stress, Anti-fatigue

Budgeting your energy by managing your emotional and physiological motors requires a targeted diet and plenty of downtime for relaxing.

MAGNESIUM IS OPTIMUM

A key element for the transformation of energy and required for more than 300 biochemical reactions, magnesium is critical for the balance of the nervous and muscular systems. **Stress saps our reserves** of magnesium, and its deficiency is one of the main causes of fatigue. Foods rich in magnesium include fruits and vegetables, especially dried ones; whole grains; and cocoa. A magnesium supplement taken at the change of seasons is recommended by many nutritionists.

Some plants can help regulate your appetite for graceful aging. **Guarana**, a physical and mental stimulant, slows digestion and helps to burn fats. **Caralluma** regulates the feeling of fullness, stimulates basic metabolism, and eases problems for people who have a tendency for compulsive eating.

SUGAR LEADS TO SUGAR

and that's not the best fuel for energy...

Insulin is secreted by the pancreas to allow the entrance of blood glucose into the cells. A high level of insulin accelerates aging. You reduce it by avoiding sugar so as not to stimulate its secretion. This seems obvious, but, unfortunately, it's not quite so simple: the glycemic index (GI) of a food (its capacity to increase sugar in the blood) depends a great deal on the other components of the meal. Refined grains—white bread, mashed potatoes—are hyperglycemic. Introduce more low-GI foods into your diet, including vegetables (dried and rich in fiber), brown rice, and whole grains. Of course, your meal should have variety and be balanced and colorful. And to keep your youthful beauty, no nibbling on sweets!

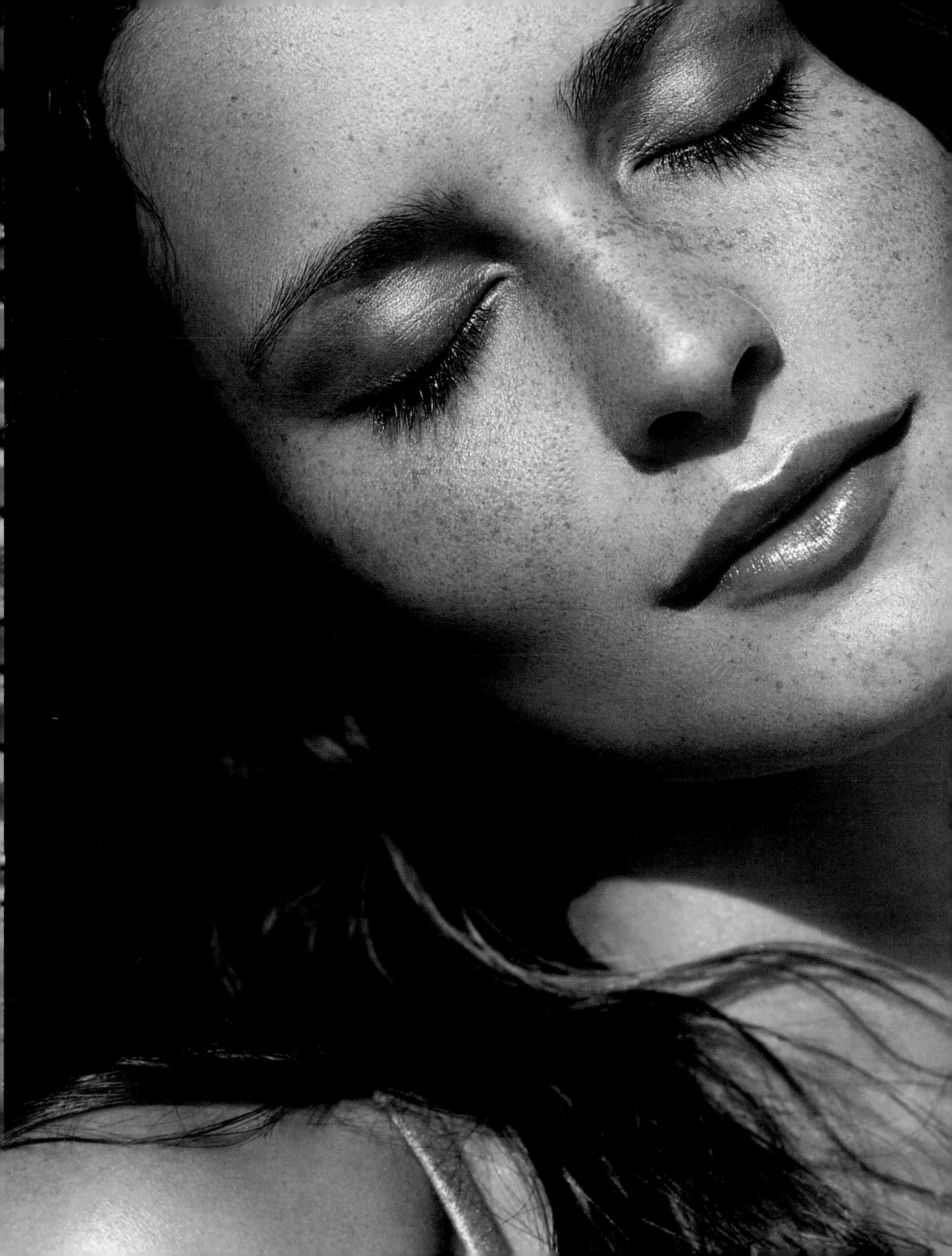

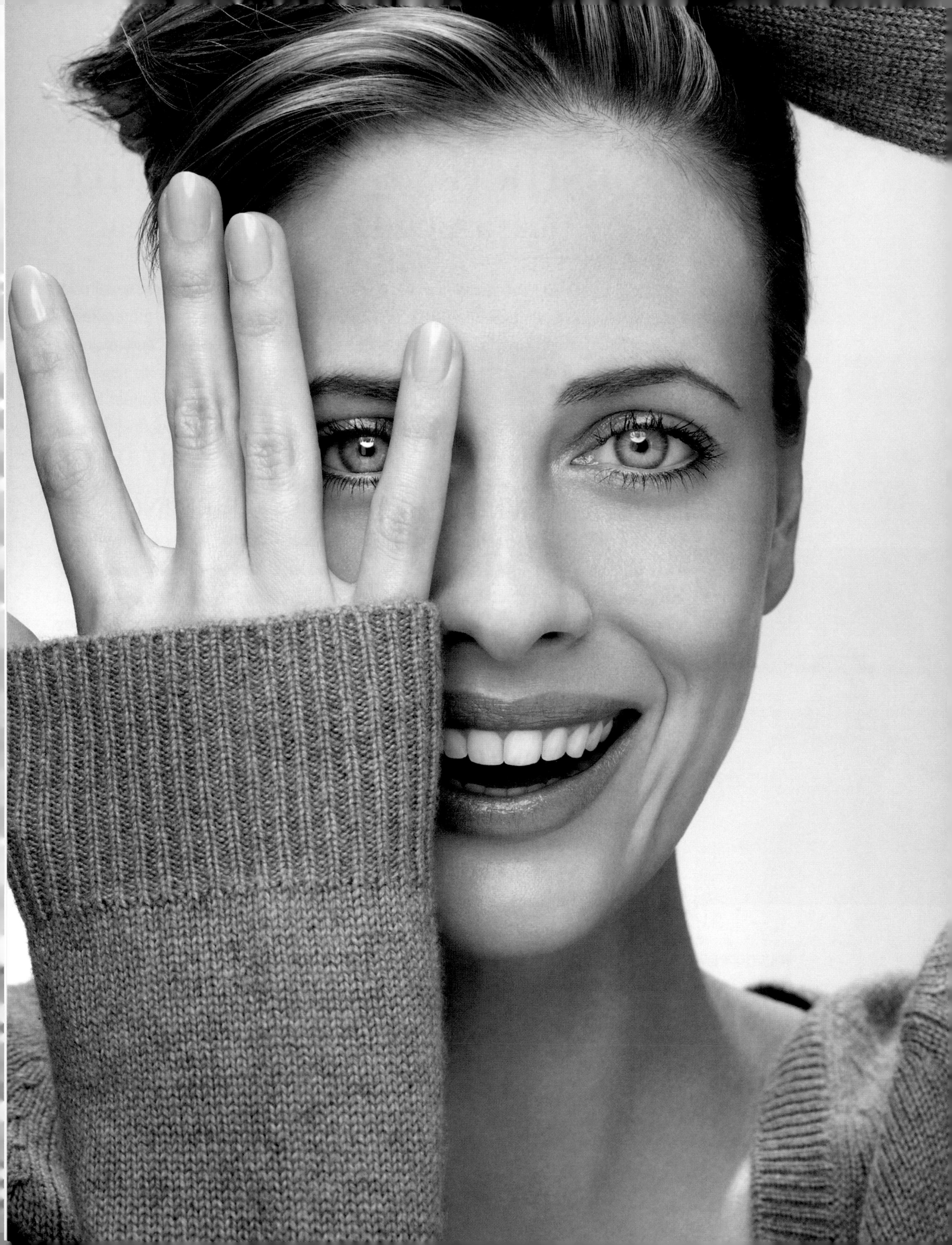

"Even a simple procedure can change your behavior and make you smile more and look more attractive."

Cosmetics can prevent, stimulate, optimize, and provide elements that will nourish and preserve your beauty—but it doesn't allow us to go back in time. Where there is a loss of material, only a true electroshock to your skin would be able to restart the process. The cells will defend themselves and once again fabricate elastin and collagen—this is what happens, for example, when skin is scarred from a burn.

The field of cosmetics is becoming closer and closer to pharmacology, and this seems to be a natural progression since we find very active molecules in plants. In optimal concentrations, we find active ingredients but no undesirable molecules.

ADVICE FROM PHARMACIST BRIGITTE LEROUX

Active dermatological ingredients are perhaps the biggest step that cosmetics has taken, with hydroxy acids (the new generations are even tolerated by those with sensitive skin) proving themselves in many medical instances and cutting-edge research. The latest active ingredients that have proved effective are salicylic acid from willow trees, glycolic acid from cane sugar, and lactic acid from tomato juice. Flavonoids and tannins, with their excellent anti-aging properties that stimulate the fundamental cells of the dermis, are also widely used.

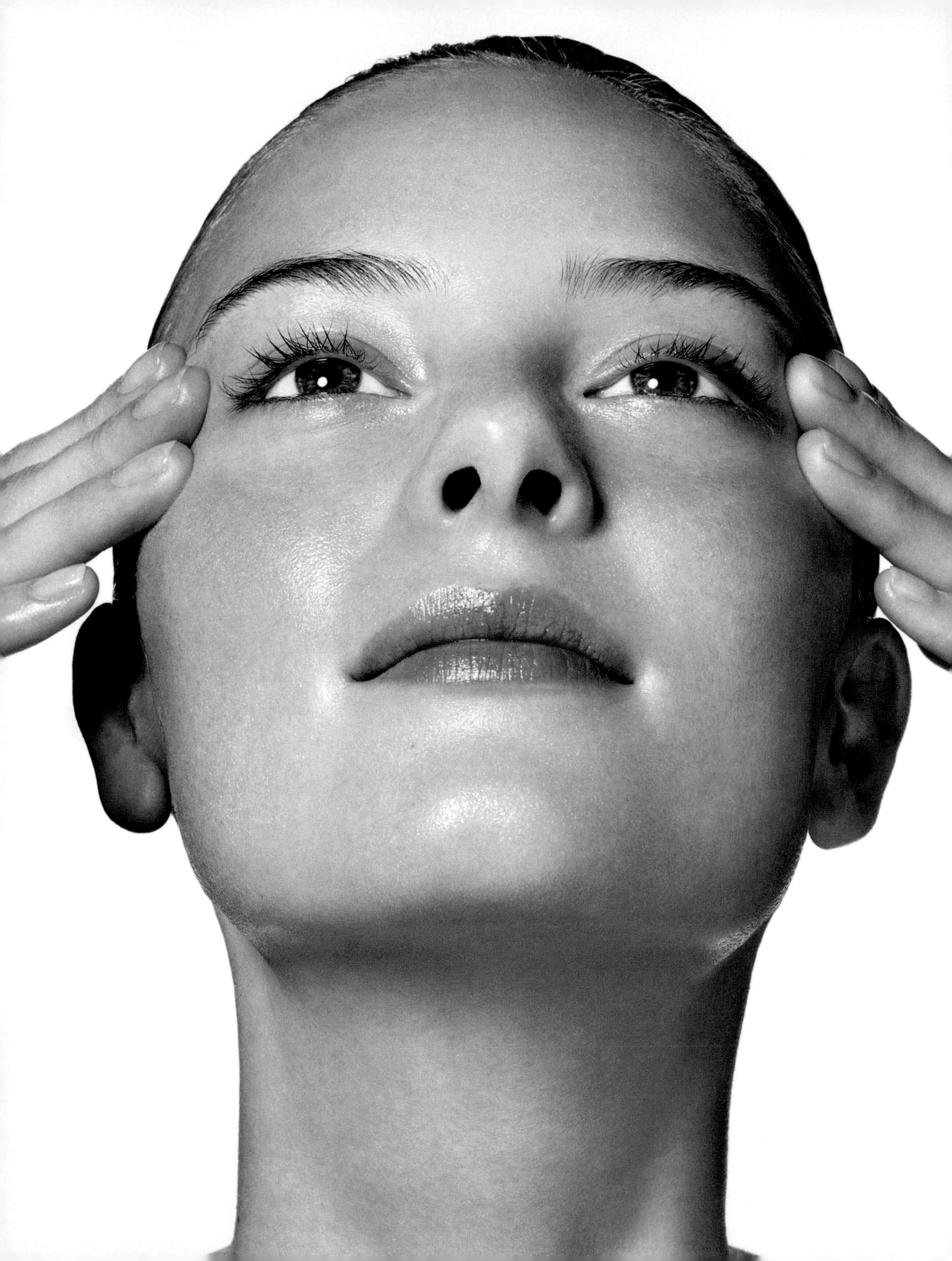

Techniques for younger skin

The progress and advancement of plastic surgery today now allow very natural results—when performed by a skilled doctor in moderation.

FOR BRIGHTER, FRESHER SKIN

When skin loses its freshness, you need to act on its overall quality to eliminate any uneven skin tone or creased appearance. Unlike filling in wrinkles, you don't treat one specific area, but the entire surface. These techniques stimulate the epidermis and the dermis, and the result is luminous skin that is more dense, more invigorated, and simply looks more beautiful!

- **Chemical peels** eliminate the dead layers of skin. The most superficial peels, based on fruit acids, do not reach the corneal layer. But the deeper peels, with trichloroacetic acid (TCA) and phenols and used under anesthesia, go as deep as the dermis. This exfoliation burns away dead tissue; the chemical shock, felt in the fibroblasts in a deep peel, reactivates cellular synthesis. Collagen and elastin fibers, as well as hyaluronic acid, hydrate and tighten the dermis. Microcirculation is visible in the softened skin, which is cleaner, tighter, and brighter. This provides true revitalization that almost erases wrinkles when the treatment is with phenols.
- **Intense pulse light (IPL)** is a technique using a laser that works wonderfully on brown spots and aging due to sun exposure, resulting in a more uniform skin tone. It also provides a kick start for collagen production.
- **Revitalization (Mesolift)** is a treatment using nonreticulated hyaluronic acid or a blend of hyaluronic acid, vitamins, and minerals that is absorbed into the epidermis and dermis. The objective is to increase the capture of water molecules in the skin (giving it a hydrophilic property), and it is targeted on the cheeks, décolletage, and hands.
- **Stimulation using radio frequency (RF)** boosts collagen production. ▶

▶ FOR BETTER SKIN TONE

Improve the structure of skin by combatting the loosening of tissue that causes faces to grow thinner, contours to fade, and cheekbones to become less prominent.

Injectables add volume by filling in thinned-out areas.

Thermal treatment, a new technique using unipolar radio frequency, denatures or modifies the molecular structure of skin via a thermal effect on the tissue to create a new source of collagen fibers. This is a way to approach sagging skin without undergoing surgery, even if it's just a temporary fix. Skin is firmer and more energized.

Lipofilling surgery remodels the face using self-transplants of fatty cells.

For Erasing Wrinkles

Here too, we use injections of products to fill in. The results are more natural because the products are gentler, injected almost painlessly into the nasogenian fold and the peribuccal region around the cheek, between the eyebrows, and at the crow's-feet. A treatment, if it is well maintained, will take years to gradually fade.

• **Hyaluronic acid** allows a beneficial balance of hydration in the skin by retaining the water it holds, but which diminishes as we age. The injections will give back volume and help to counterbalance the fragility of the skin.

• The effect will gradually fade over the course of time (9 to12 months). The injections also make up for the loss of natural collagen, whose cohesion is altered by time, allowing lines and wrinkles to appear.

Collagen-based injections cultivated under strict laboratory control (stem cells of human or pig origin) that are organic and dermatologically compatible do not require preliminary tests. The results last 6 to 12 months.

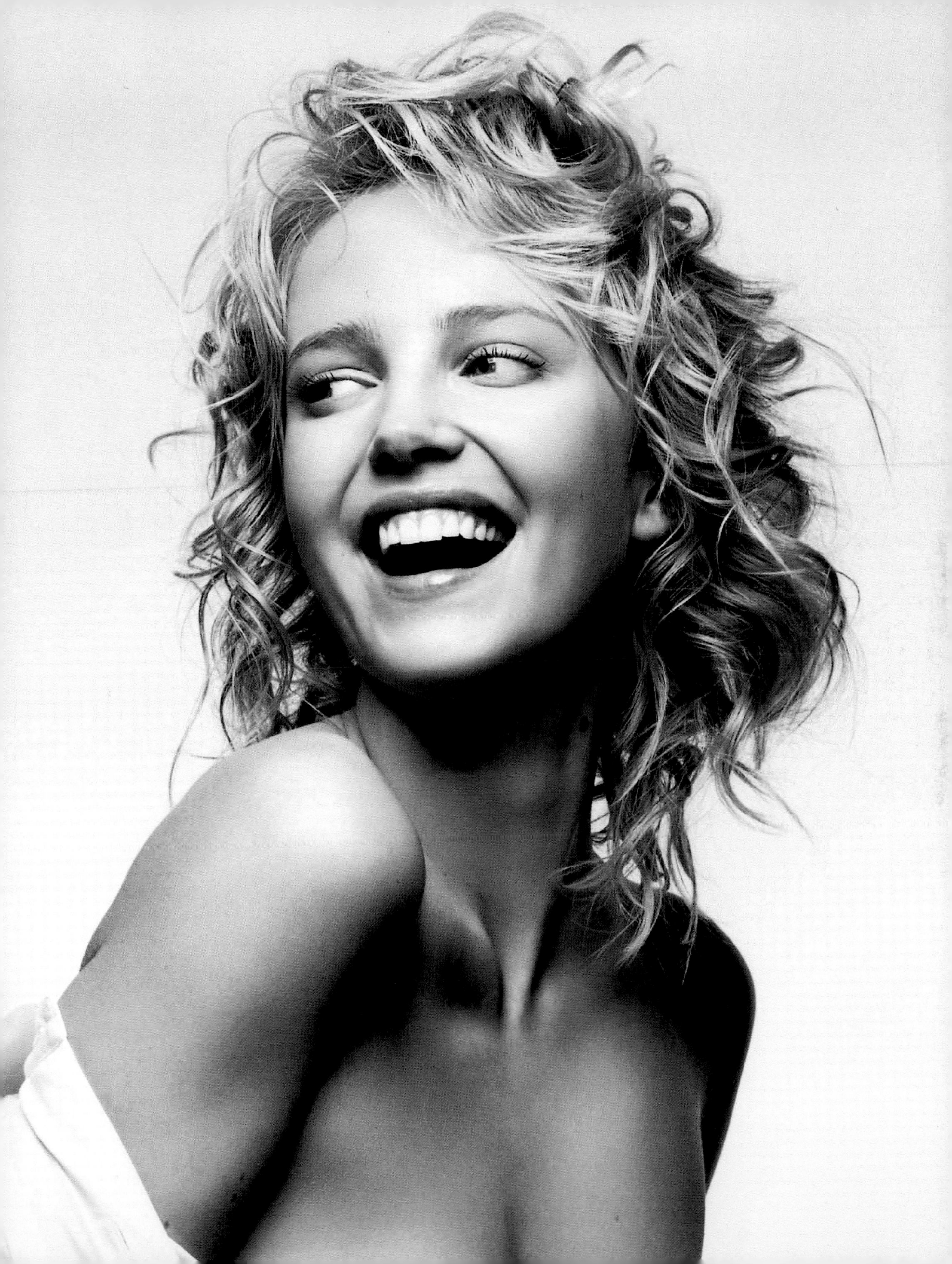

Plan your time to save yourself from the passage of time

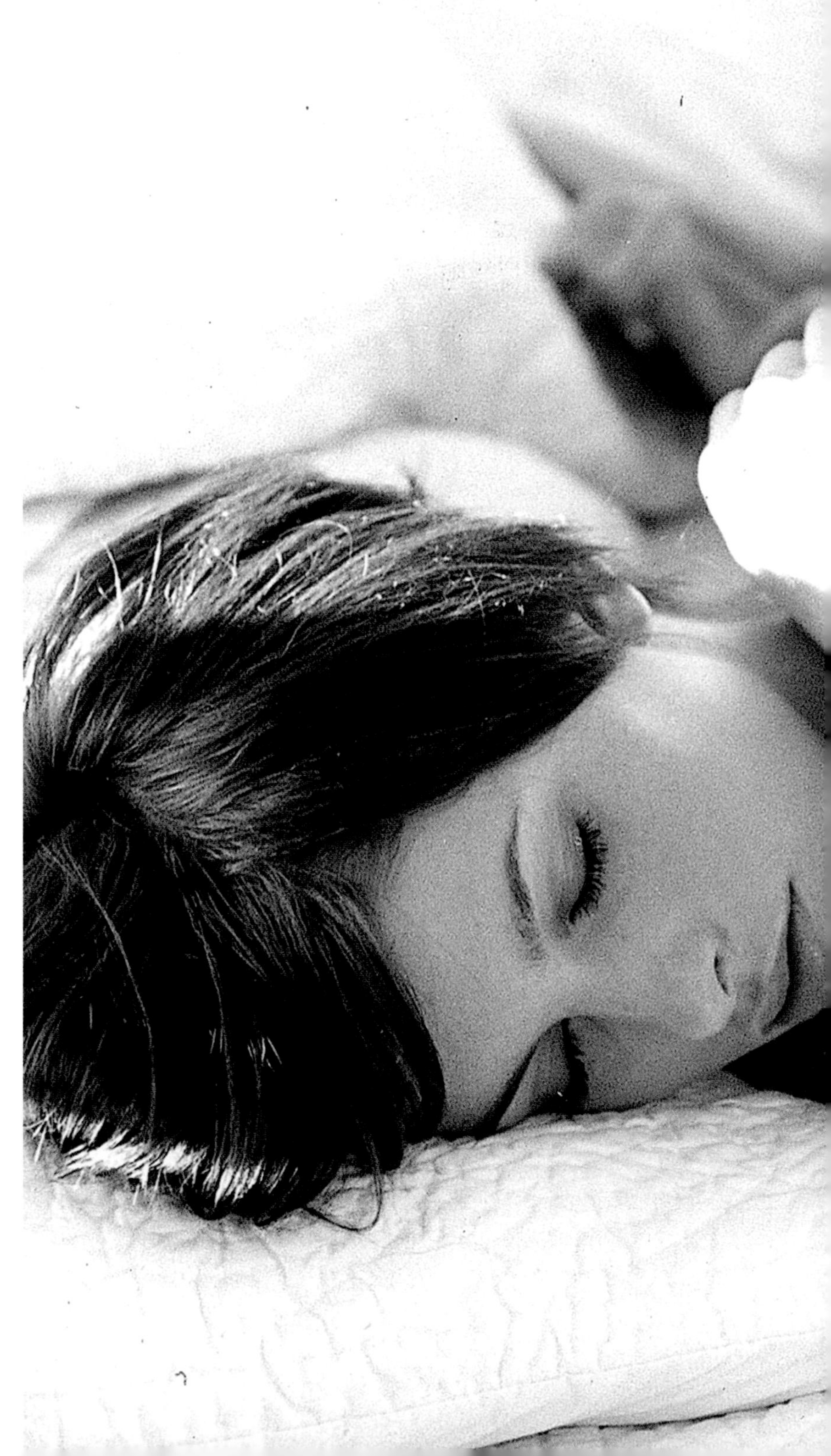

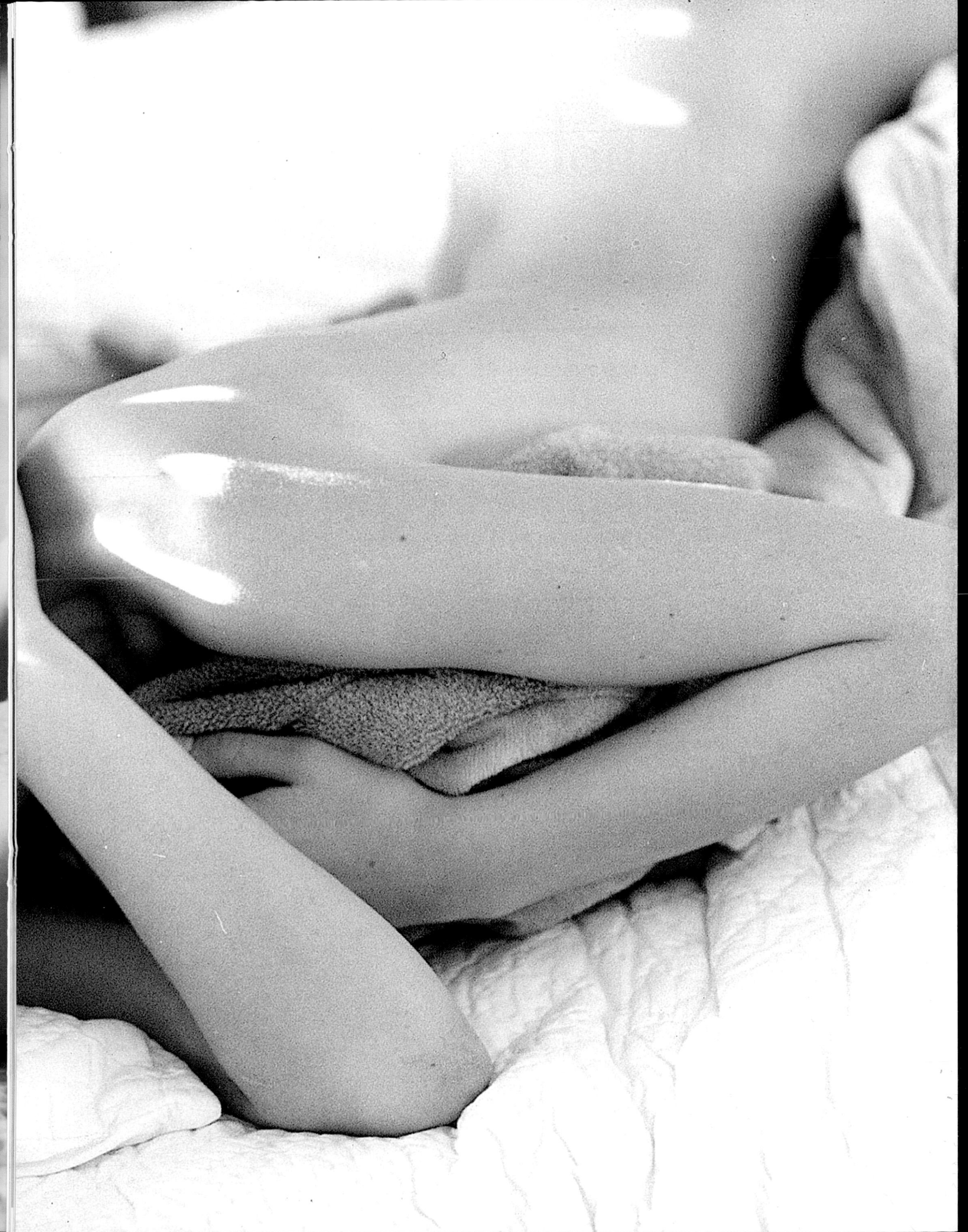

Qigong, Tai Chi: meditation with Benefits

A trend from the East, these disciplines rebalance the body's energies with a preventive approach inspired by Chinese medicine and acupuncture. Why not take a class and discover their powers?

QIGONG: DETOX WORKOUT

Slowness is elevated to the level of fine art with this energy work inspired by Chinese medicine and Taoism. Similar to acupuncture, it heals the body by reestablishing the **flow of vital energy (qi)** through pressure points. It's a very gentle combination of movements made during intense concentration, breathing, and massage and has a beneficial impact on the entire body, including the organs responsible for eliminating wastes. Of course, the prospect of **discovering the eight treasures** or **soaring like a purple swallow** is motivation enough.

TAI CHI: RELAXING BOXING

Tai chi is a return to the ancient **art of shadow boxing** against your own shadow zones, and this martial art, practiced by Buddhist monks, has found a new following. Transmuted into slow exercise with a gracefully timed series of flowing movements, it takes gentle care of your mental health as well as the health of your muscles. Tai chi increases your powers of concentration and is based on extremely relaxing movements that stimulate the nervous system and blood circulation. Invigorated by a warm current, you feel a real energy, which helps to manage stress and overactivity, and a wholeness, which gives confidence in your own abilities.

Done first thing in the morning, qigong and tai chi, based on a preventive aspect that provides control over the flow of energies, are very harmonious ways to start the day.

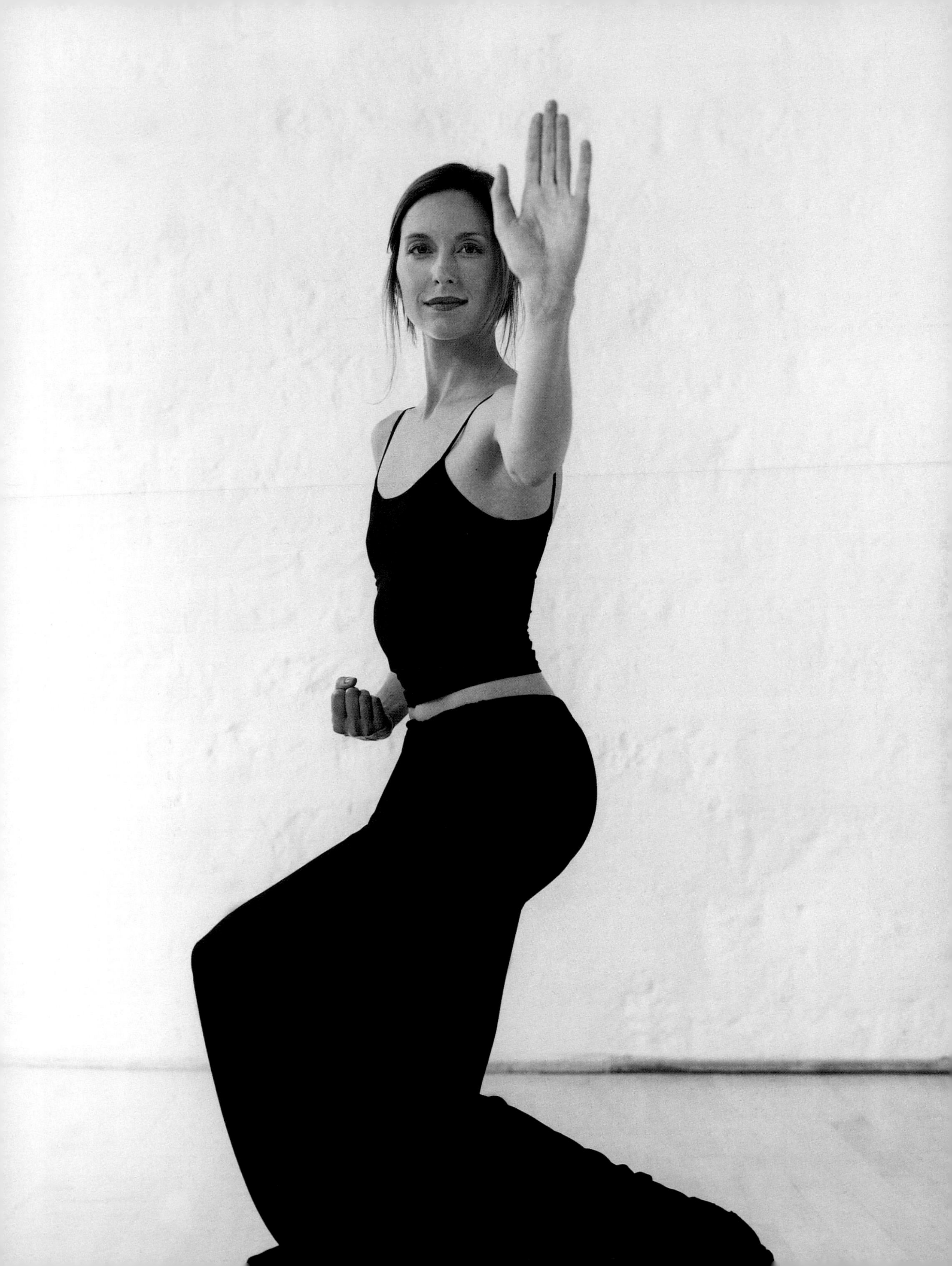

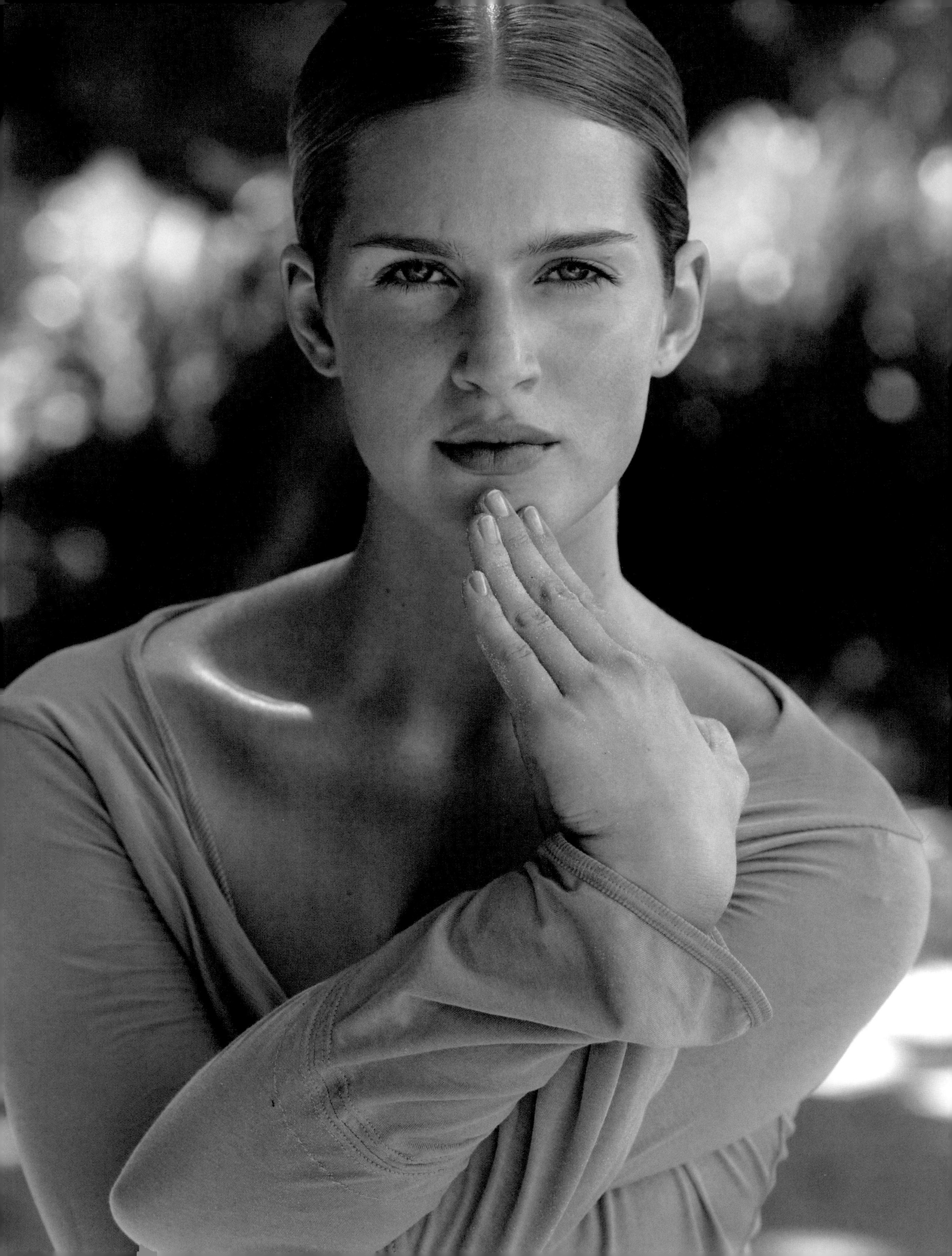

Gentle energy

Move smoothly and get some fresh air without losing your breath. Here's a quick lesson on how to get in shape without breaking a sweat!

INSPIRED BY YOGA, this is a brief session of gentle stretching practiced while breathing deeply.

1 **STRETCH** With your arms outstretched and back straight, make fencing-type lunges on your right leg and then your left.

2 **LOOSEN UP** Keeping your spine straight, pivot at your waist. Place the left hand on the left foot and then the right hand on the right foot. Then place your right hand on your left foot and your left hand on your right foot.

3 **BEND** With your spine straight, arms straight above you, and palms together, bend at the waist to your right and then to your left.

4 **BECOME MORE FLEXIBLE** Seated, bend at the waist toward your feet and grasp them at your toes. Keeping your legs straight in front of you, lean back on your buttocks.

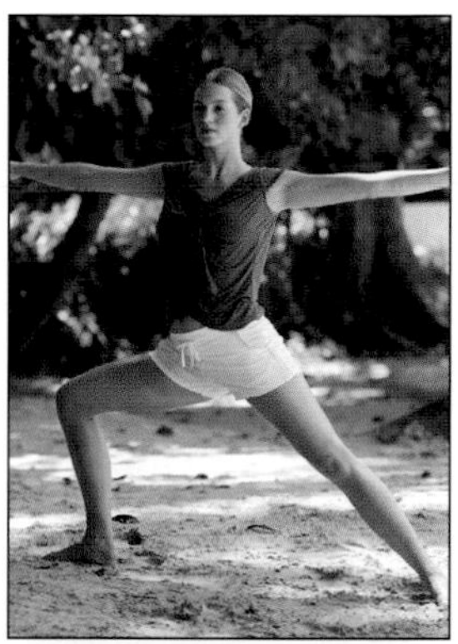
1

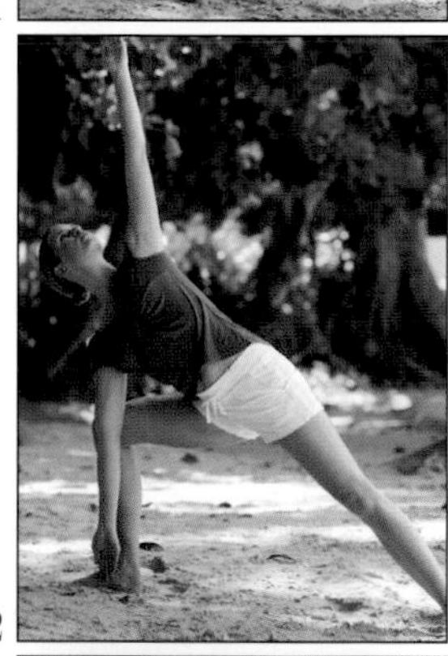
2

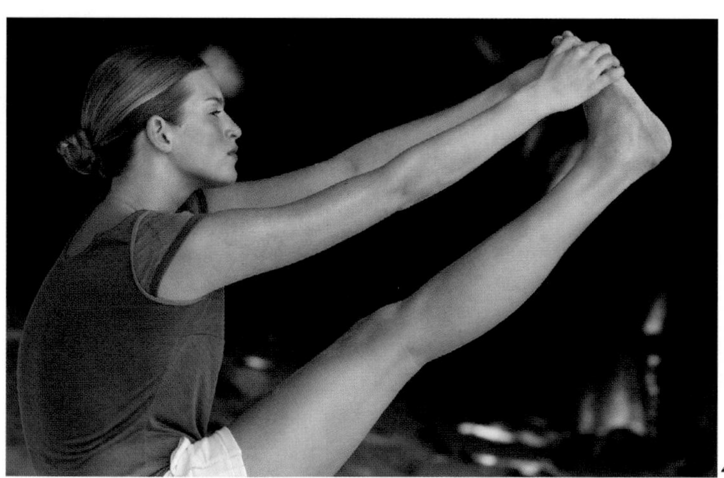
4

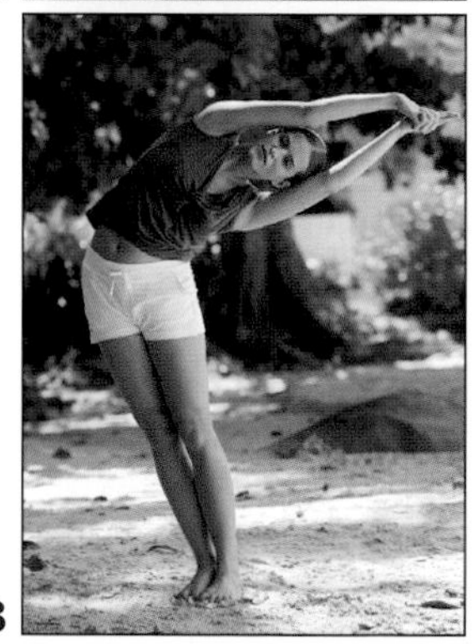
3

Two styles of exercise

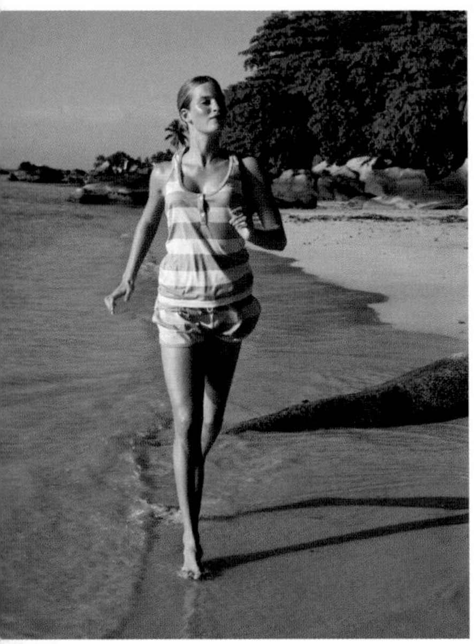

Walk in the water! The ideal depth is right to the knee. Providing the freshness of a massage, you build on the effects of walking and water therapy for the ankles and calves, for perfectly shapely legs.

You don't need beautiful turquoise water and miles of gorgeous beaches for the daily practice of two perfect sports: swimming and walking!

SWIMMING

Swimming is the **perfect sport** to give you a **well-toned body.** There is less risk of injury than while running: you're in a state of weightlessness, without tension on your ligaments; you soften your lumbar vertebrae; you learn how to breathe properly; you reinforce your cardiovascular potential by boosting your circulation; and you benefit from a total-body massage.

Every swimming stroke has its purpose. Choose the ones that are best for your morphology. They all showcase the long muscles: they tone the arms (triceps especially), develop the torso, firm the chest, and reinforce the back. The **crawl** sculpts shoulders, the **breaststroke** tones the inner thighs, the **sidestroke** thins the waist, and the **backstroke** yields a beautiful back. Taking a few classes to learn these strokes would be useful and would help you benefit most from your workout.

WALKING

Taking advantage of every opportunity to walk remains the best elixir for life (especially for people who cannot play sports). It's an option available to everyone, city dwellers included, to skip the car or leave for the metro station a bit earlier. Not only will you see the benefits in your figure but you'll also improve your circulation, encourage digestion, provide oxygen to the body, and slow osteoporosis. Moreover, a solitary walk helps concentration and allows you to make good decisions. It's the easiest mental and physical detox cure.

ADVICE FROM AN ANGIOLOGIST

It's a question of public health! Moving is the best assurance of longevity. Ten thousand steps per day is the ideal recommendation for good health. Walking, swimming, and pedaling are perfect, but not all sports are good for the veins—for example, jumping in place (step aerobics and aerobics) and stationary machines (especially ones that use too much weight). Make the most of cardio workouts in the gym, doubles tennis, and jogging on soft terrain (three miles maximum).

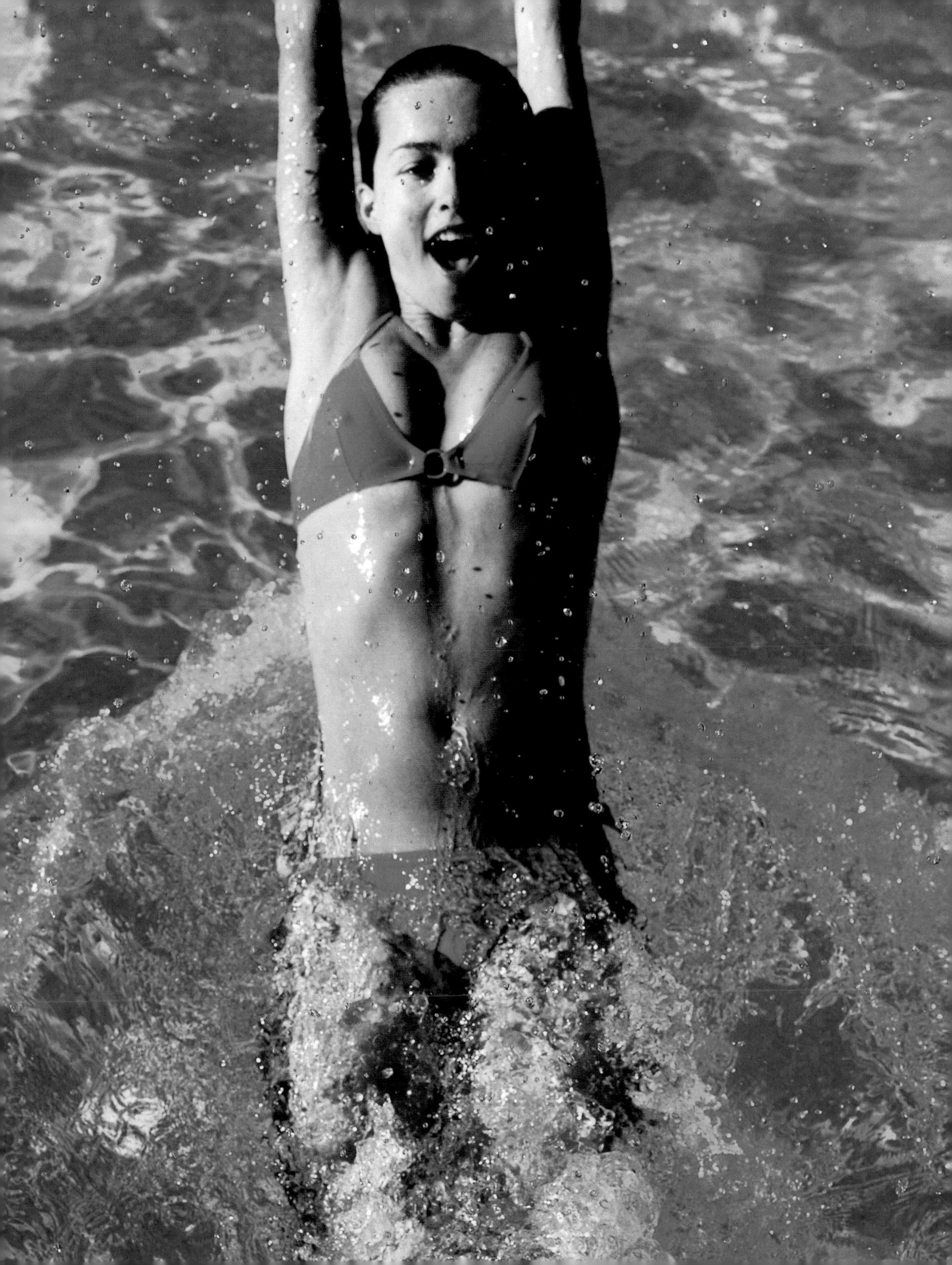

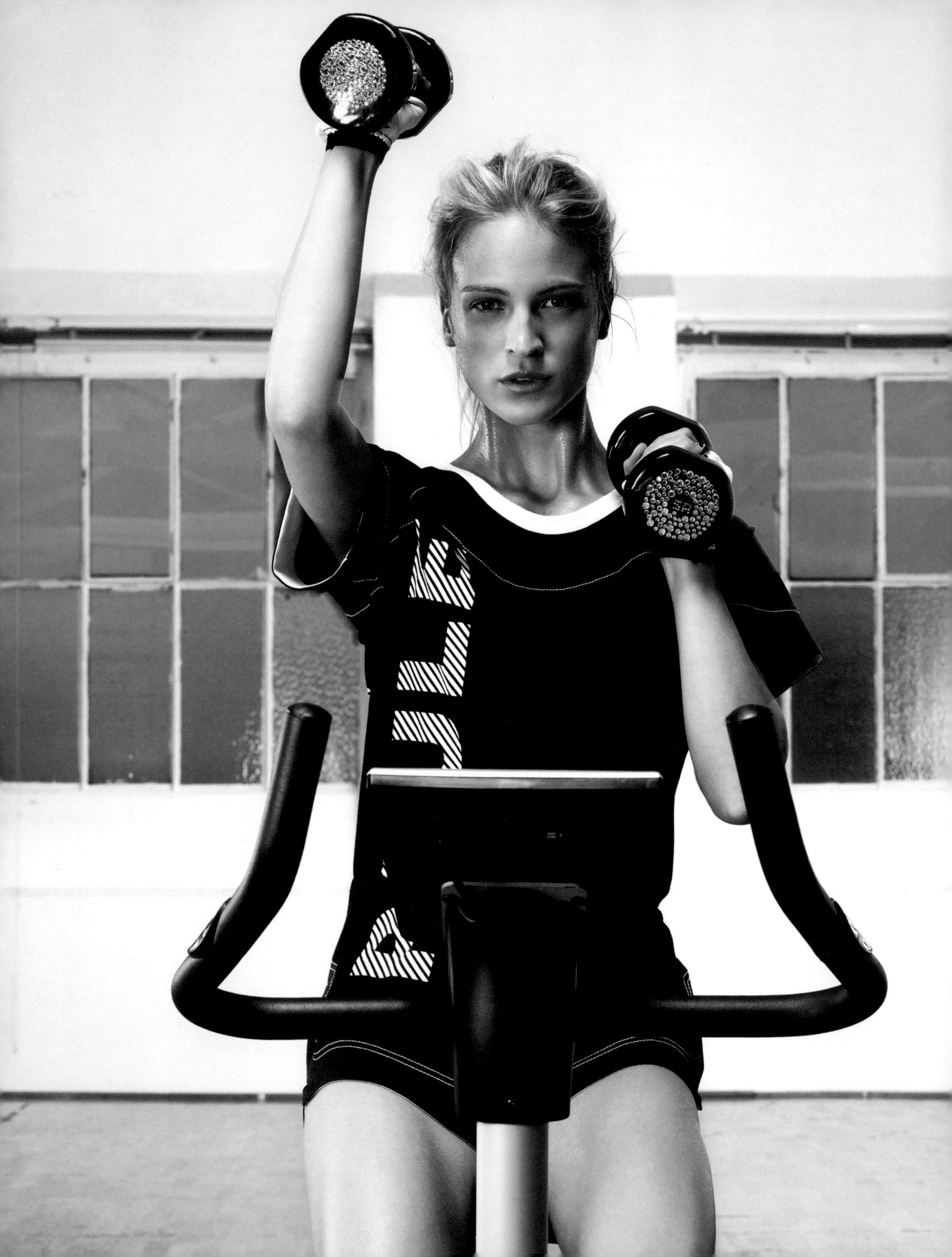

Body sculpting: work out at the gym

These tools offer endlessly innovative ways to sculpt your body into one of an athlete and boost your morale by attracting everyone's attention!

1 **STATIONARY BIKE** A very athletic device, the stationary bike provides an intense cardiovascular workout while toning your buttocks and thighs. In the course of the workout, which alternates periods of speed with pauses to catch your breath, add small dumbbells once the core of your body is warmed up to complete the cardio effect. Work the arms while you pedal, moving your back muscles, deltoids, and triceps.

This is perfect if you want a low impact sport.

2 **SISMO FITNESS:** It does (almost) everything for you! This is a fantastic machine since the oscillations practically replace the effort of your muscles. The gyrating effect from front to back and left to right (the seesaw effect is even more pronounced the more you spread your feet apart) mobilizes the deep muscle tissue (which a traditional workout does not do), activates blood circulation and lymphatic flow, and in 10 minutes gives the equivalent of one hour of working out. There are four basic positions depending on the targeted areas of the body (in the photo, with knees slightly bent, you work your thighs and calves).

This is perfect if you hate working out, are overweight, or have back or joint problems. 2 ▶

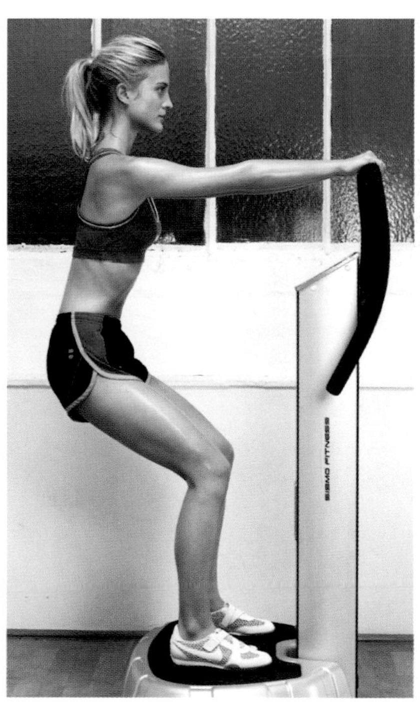

Building tone and muscle, providing a new momentum, and sculpting the perfect abs.

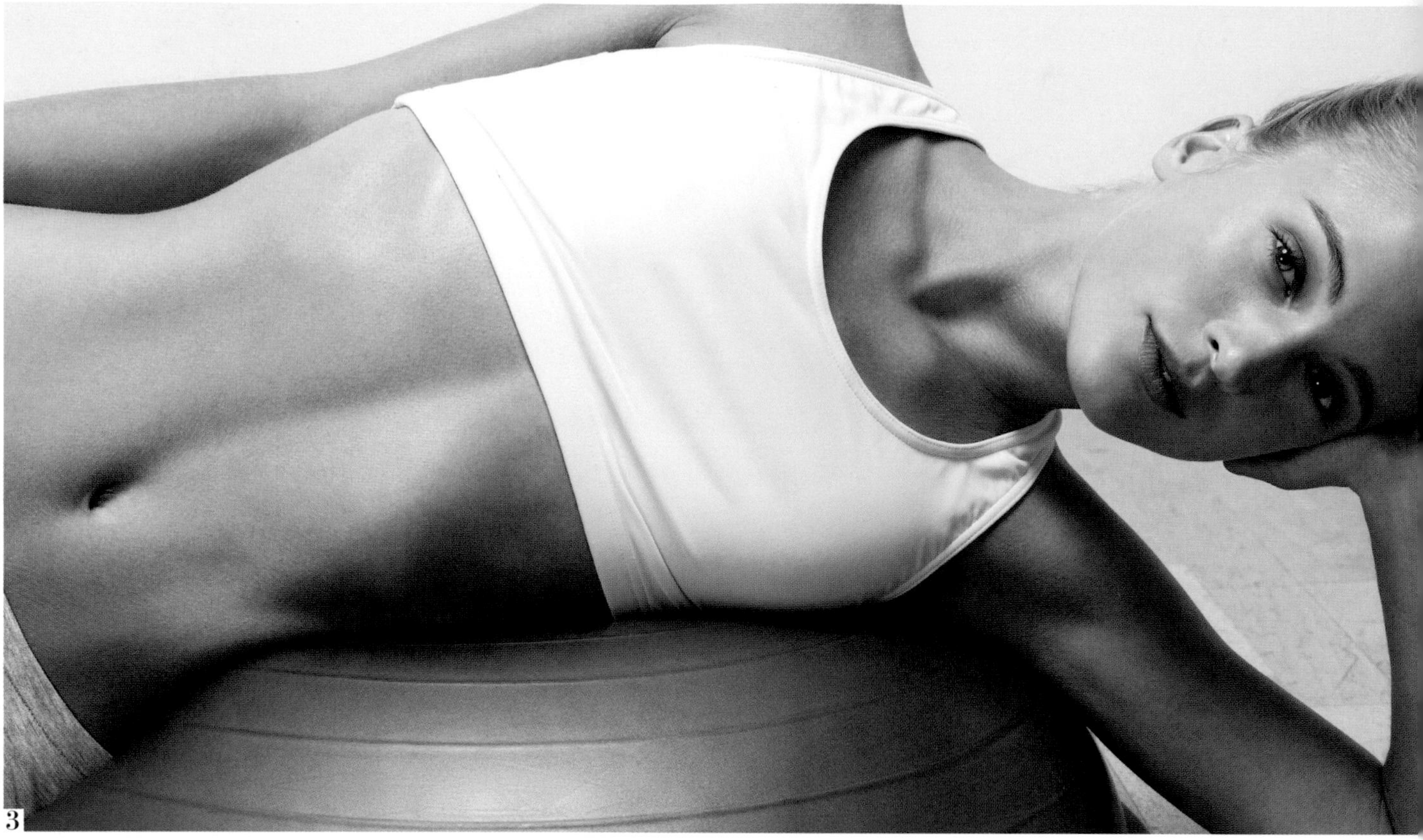

3

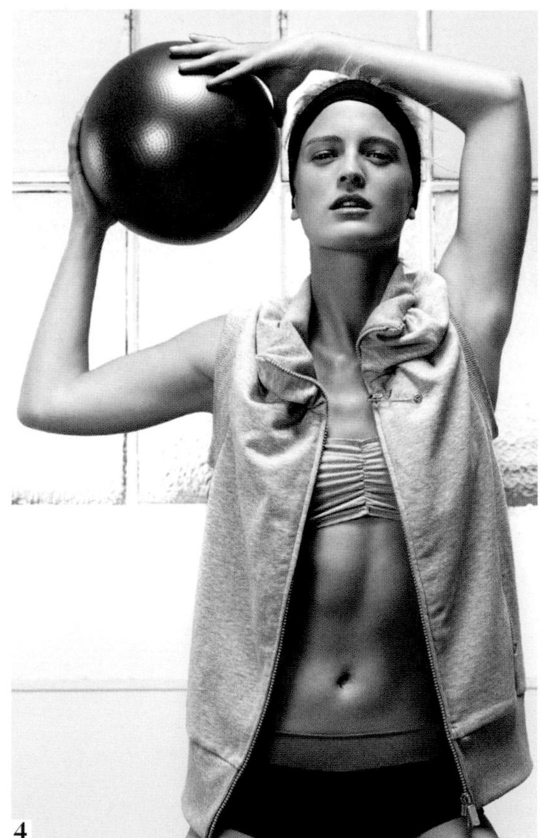

4

3 BALANCE BALL: PLAYFUL! You adapt traditional floor exercises to this soft sphere, which requires you to compensate for the imbalance by using the core muscles that provide the foundation for your chest and spine. The result: a firmer, thinner waist. Have fun while you reap the benefits!

4 BODYVIVE: SOFTBALL WORKOUT Ideal for a more gentle workout, Bodyvive, based on a series of movements and choreography using accessories, is intended to enhance tone, mobility, endurance, and agility. This is a program developed by the athlete Les Mills, the father of group exercise, and uses balls, elastic bands, and dumbbells.

5 KRUMPING: TAKE YOUR BREATH AWAY! Street dancing is revisited and channeled into the classroom to sculpt abs and buttocks, while at the same time releasing energy—and even aggression—with superquick hip-hop tempos.

5

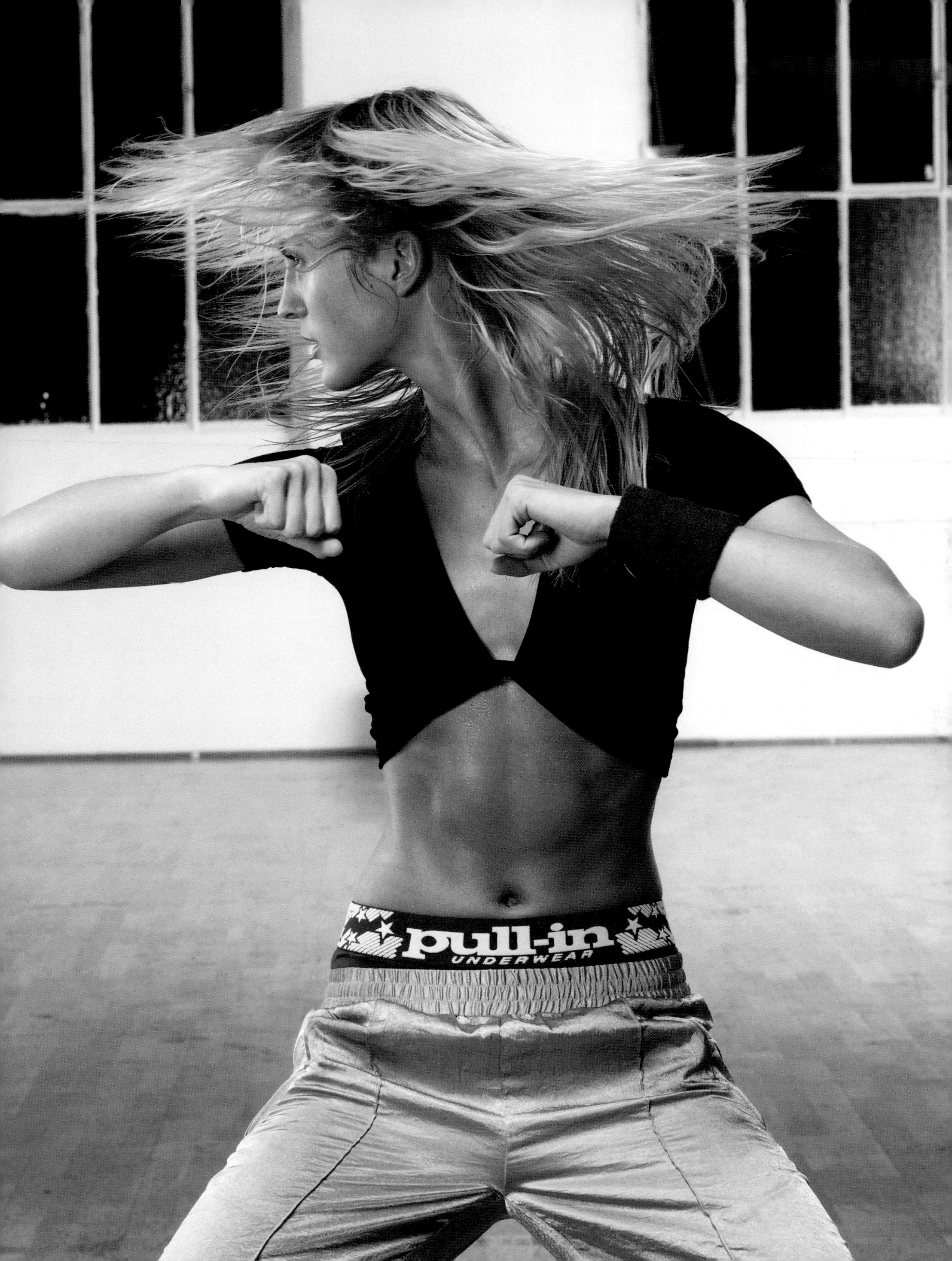
pull-in
UNDERWEAR

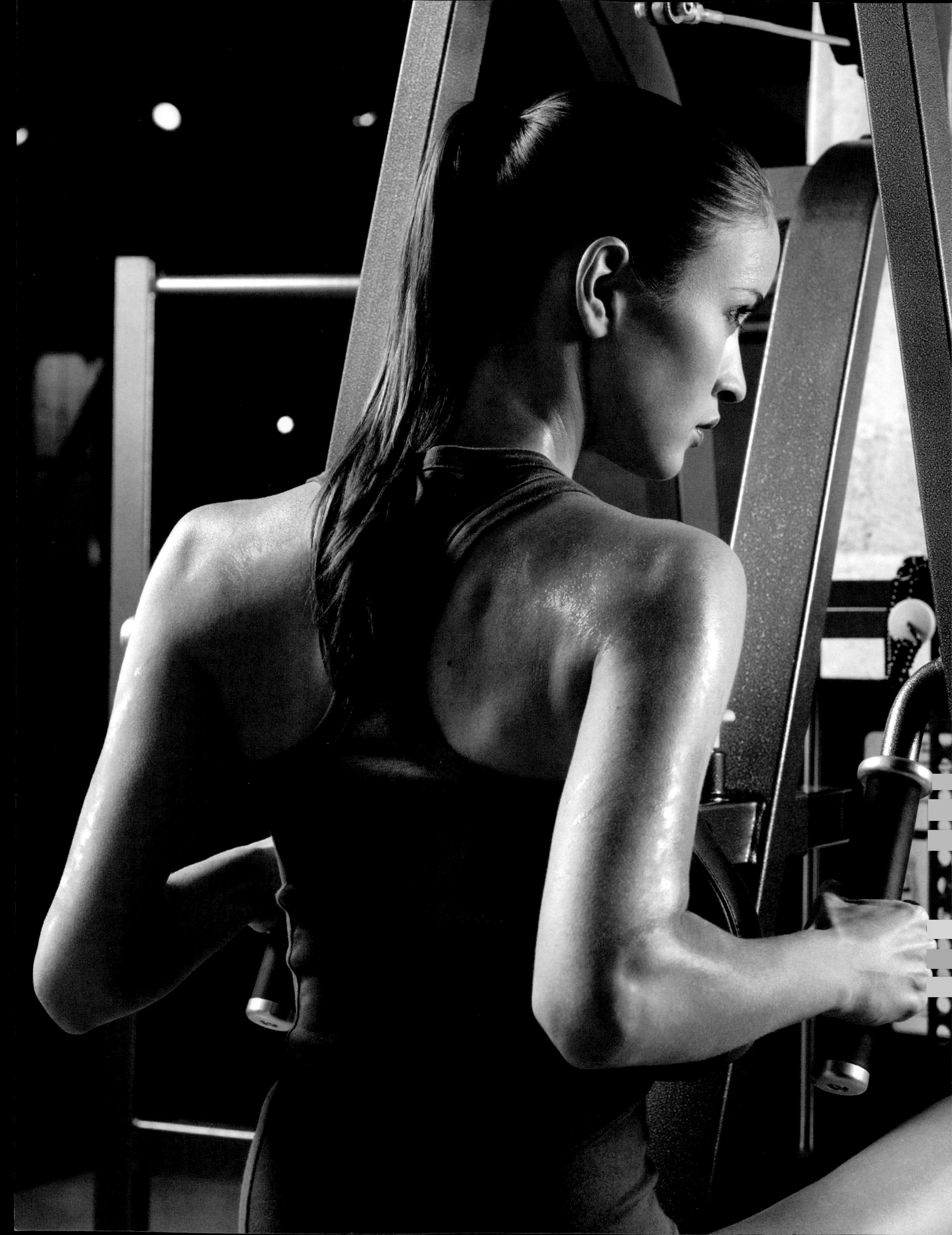

Body sculpting: using machines

These body sculpting techniques are adapted for women (and are to be practiced only under professional guidance) for ultratargeted results. A guided tour.

1 A BEAUTIFUL BACK Perfect for erasing the hours spent in front of the television with your shoulders slouched and posture far from perfect, the rowing machine works on your shoulders by opening them up and improves and maintains the muscle tone of your upper back. Sit on the bench facing the machine and push the bar horizontally until your arms are outstretched. With your arms locked at chest level, you'll intensely feel the work of your muscles spread from your shoulder blades all the way down your arms. Use this machine with moderation if you have neck problems or shoulder pain.

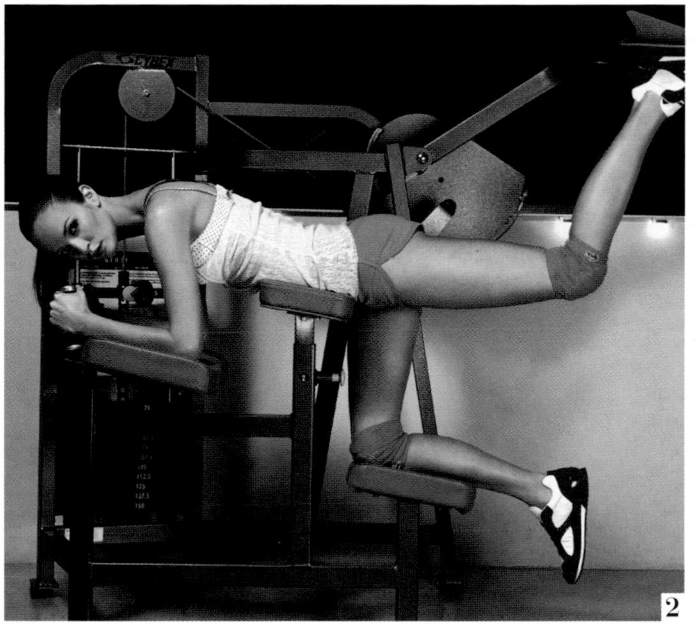
2

2 YOUR BUTTOCKS' BEST FRIEND They become incredibly firm in record time thanks to this machine, which requires you to work the gluteus maximus muscles without arching your back. You accentuate your curves while slimming the upper thighs. In a position on all fours, raise your head level with your chest and extend your spine. Then push the bar up with your leg. This is a technique reserved for abs and buttocks fanatics and truly is extremely effective.

◄1

▶

Gym workouts have evolved a great deal and have adapted to new needs by moving closer and closer to individualized attention. A personal trainer at the gym will listen to your needs and desires and will advise you on the best course of action. The pros are there to guide you every step of the way.

THE BEST IN THE WORLD

Emphasize relaxation and just let go

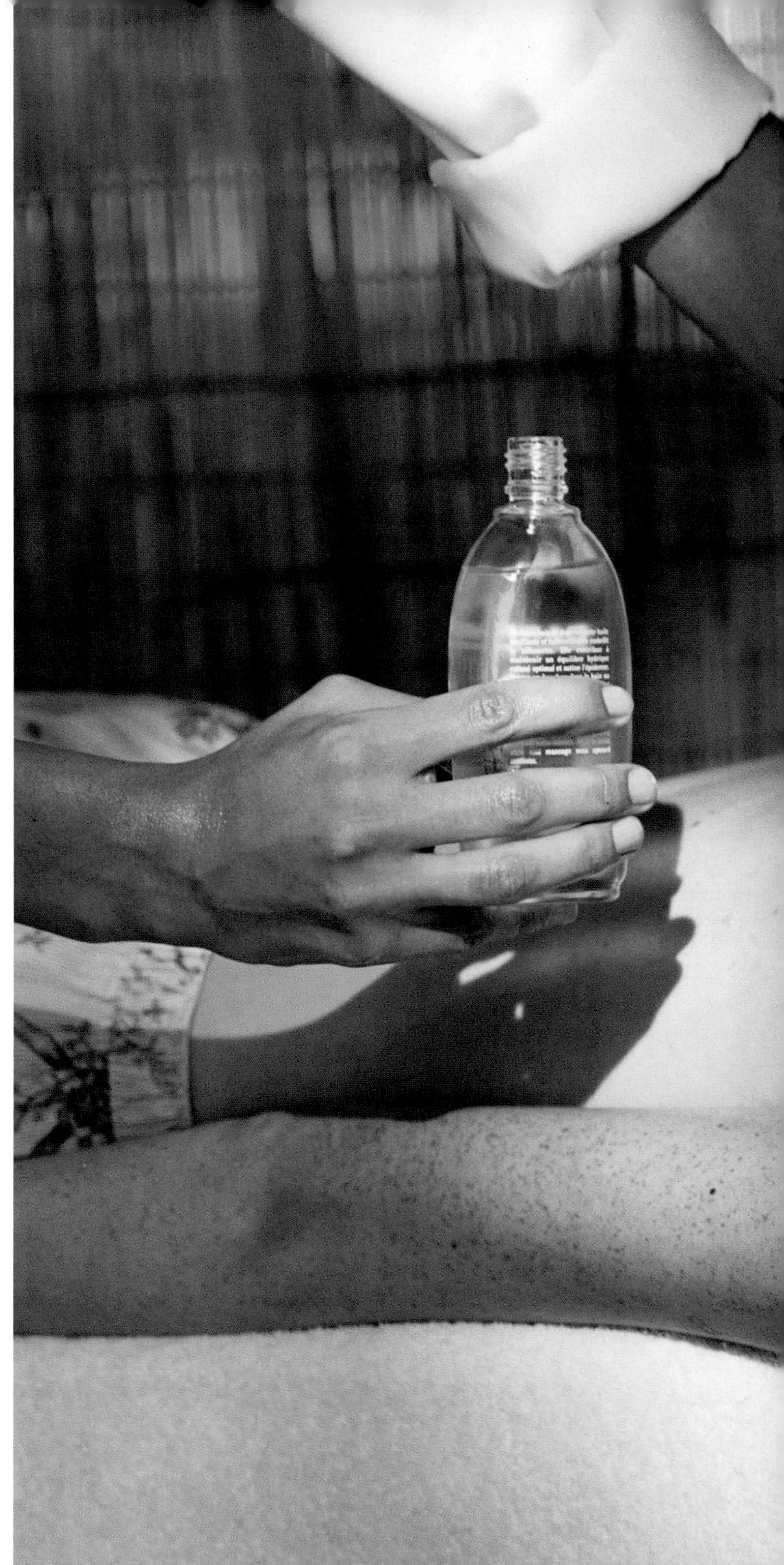

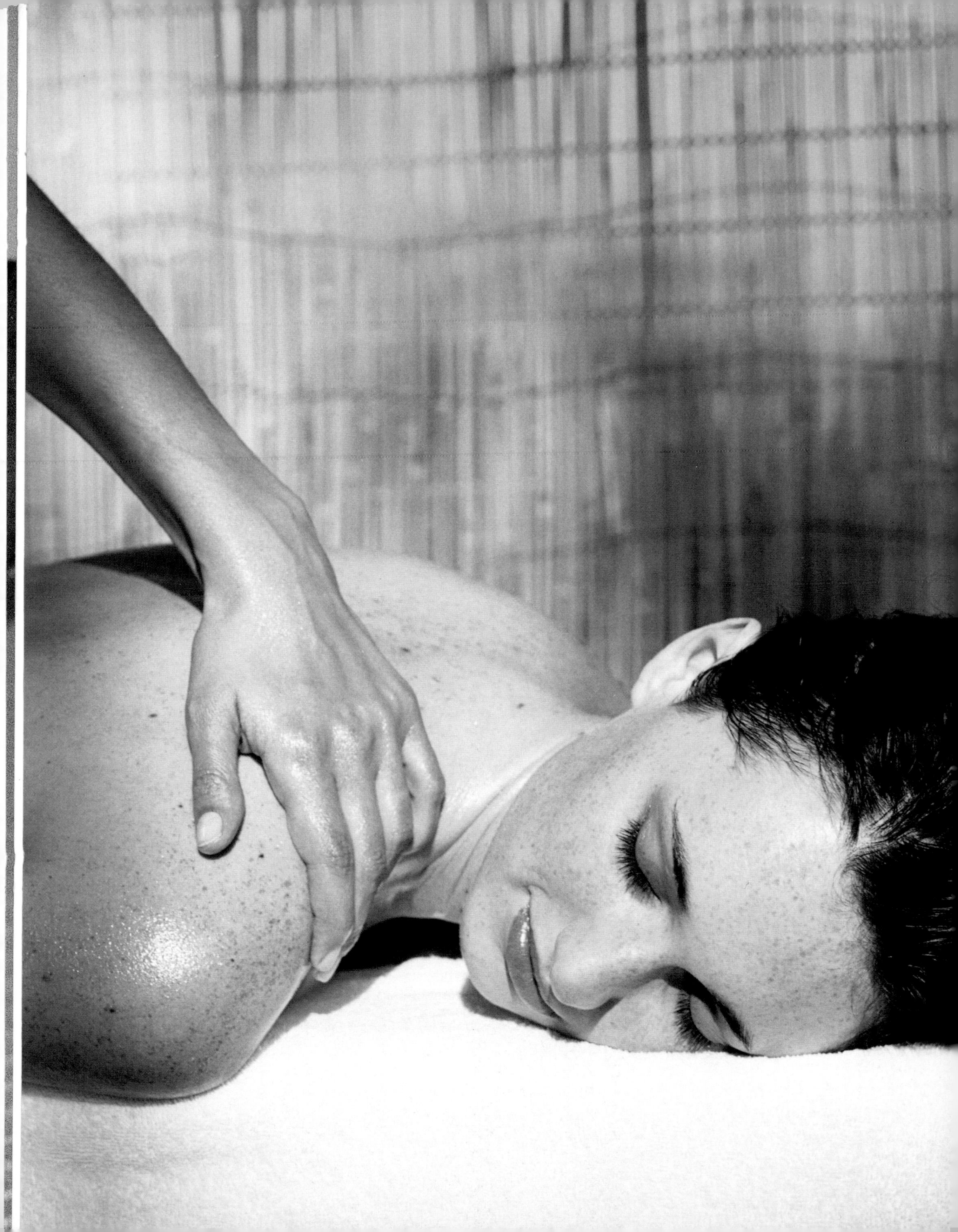

Seawater therapy

The waves of seawater therapy (thalassotherapy) are overflowing and propose a wide range of targeted treatments for relaxation and overall wellness.

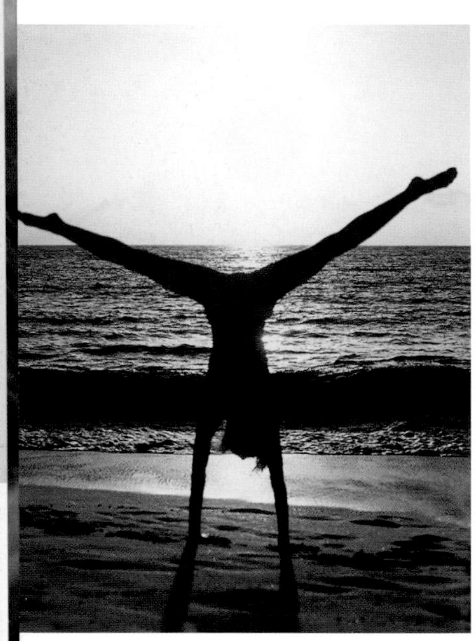

Infinitely rich, the place of our origins is full of promise and contains a great number of medications. These range from the prostaglandins in coral to the many cephalosporins, the first antibiotics from the sea, and the anticancer discoveries in the stomach of sharks or in sea sponges!

LIFE NEEDS SALT

Totally in sync with our blood plasma, seawater is a pure wonder that concentrates mineral salts, trace elements (iodine, calcium, magnesium), proteins, plankton, seaweeds, and marine clay. This is argument enough for us to take a dip! Seawater therapy offers an iodized combination of all the benefits of the ocean when performed under supervision and with a preventative or curative goal. We fill our lungs with **pure sea air, charged with ozone and ultrainvigorating negative ions,** to stimulate the blood and reinforce our defenses.

Enjoyed at a treatment facility along the coastline (which is obviously the best way), the water is heated to 93°F to facilitate penetration into the pores of the skin and goes to work on the little (and big) problems of the overall organism which has been overtaxed and exhausted by pollution and stress of every kind. Baths, jets, and showers replace the minerals, energize the body and mind, eliminate toxins, and stimulate the defenses for better vital functions. And you're invigorated like never before!

SEA ENERGY!

You can get a full-body mask, pressure therapy, hydrojets, and other new-wave treatments, as well as traditional ones linked with sports, cultural events, alternative medicine (osteopathy, aromatherapy, naturopathic), or Eastern medicine. Depending upon on the destination and its offerings, anything is possible. Among the pioneers, Roscoff and Quiberon have been around for a century with full-scale innovations such as underwater fitness machines (Carnac) and water dance (Bénodet).

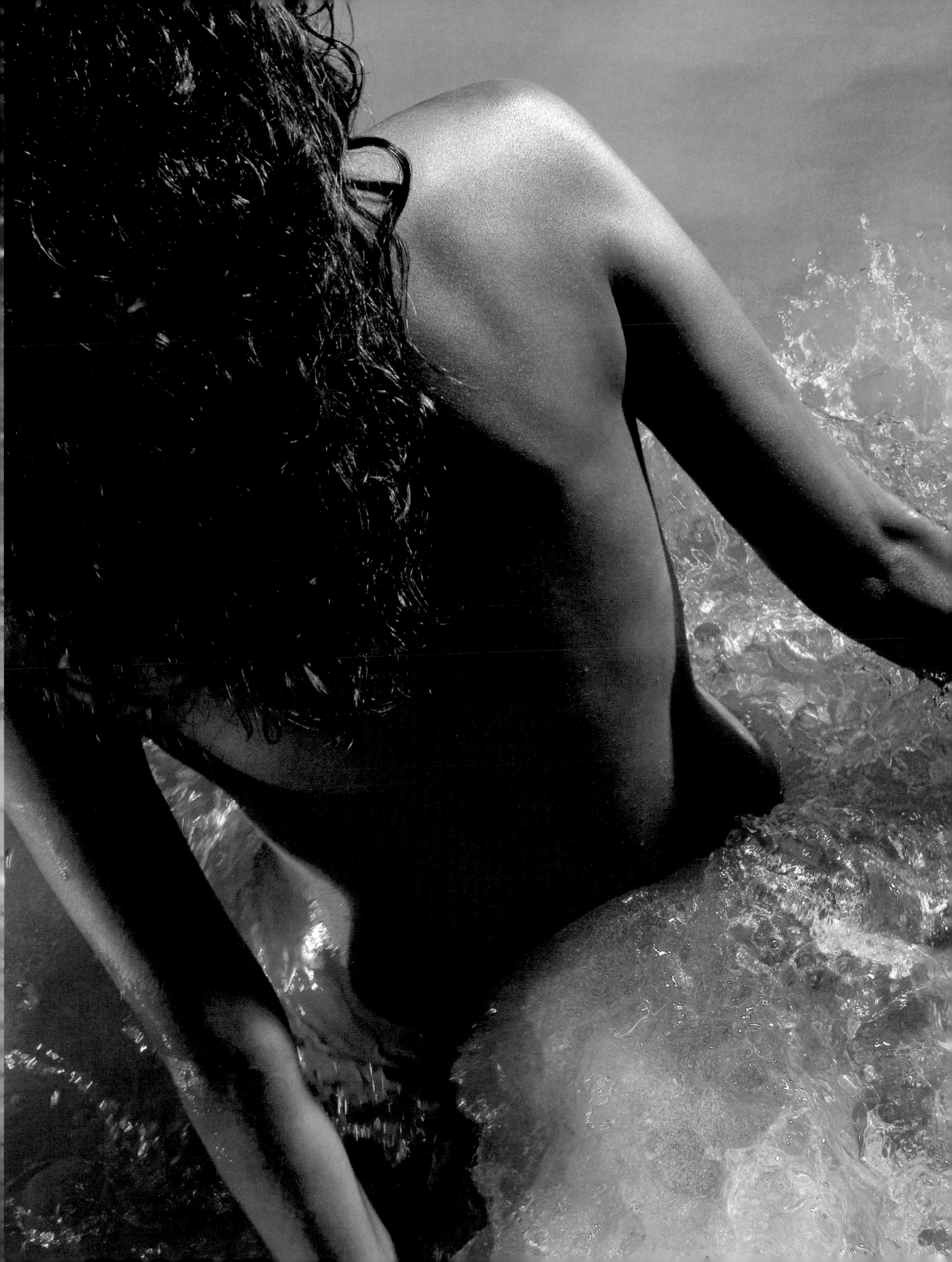

Aromatherapy: precious essential oils

Essential oils make aromatherapy one of the most refined therapies. It's an olfactory and sensual discovery, to be inhaled without moderation.

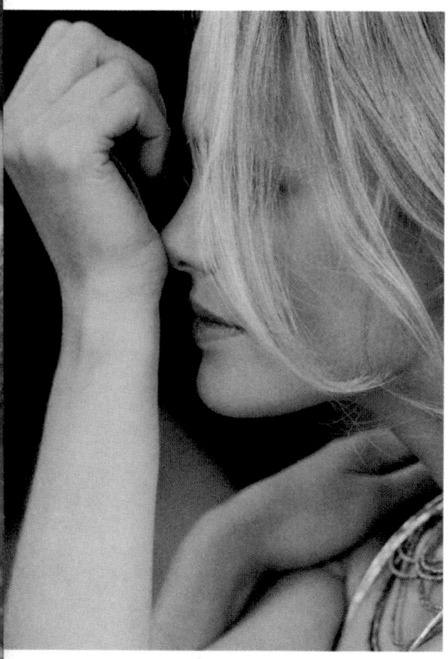

There have been no therapeutic trials to confirm the powers of aromatherapy. But, interestingly enough, a recent scientific article demonstrated the effects of perfume on the skin's immunity: an allergic reaction can sometimes be regulated with the simple inhalation of a fragrance.

INHALE HEALTH?

From insomnia to hay fever to skin problems, the applications of aromatherapy, **which is an olfactory version of herbal medicine,** are endless.

Despite their name, they are not actually oily (and unlike their vegetable cousins, they do not stain). Essential oils are steam extracted using a sophisticated and costly procedure. **Shockingly, five tons of rose petals are needed to produce a single liter of rose essence!**

40 ESSENTIAL REASONS TO IMMERSE YOURSELF IN PLEASURE

When the scent permeates the air, magnified by the warmth of a **bath** or the touch of a **massage** (mixed with almond oil, for example) or used in a **scent diffuser,** the waves of fragrance from any of the 40-odd essential oils work to improve your mood as well as your body. However, as with every active ingredient, you must use them wisely and in the correct amounts—and keep them out of reach of children.

SUPERSTAR OILS

Cypress, borage, evening primrose to improve circulation
Coriander, mint, nutmeg for energy
Eucalyptus and cinnamon to kill microbes
Cumin and mint for digestion

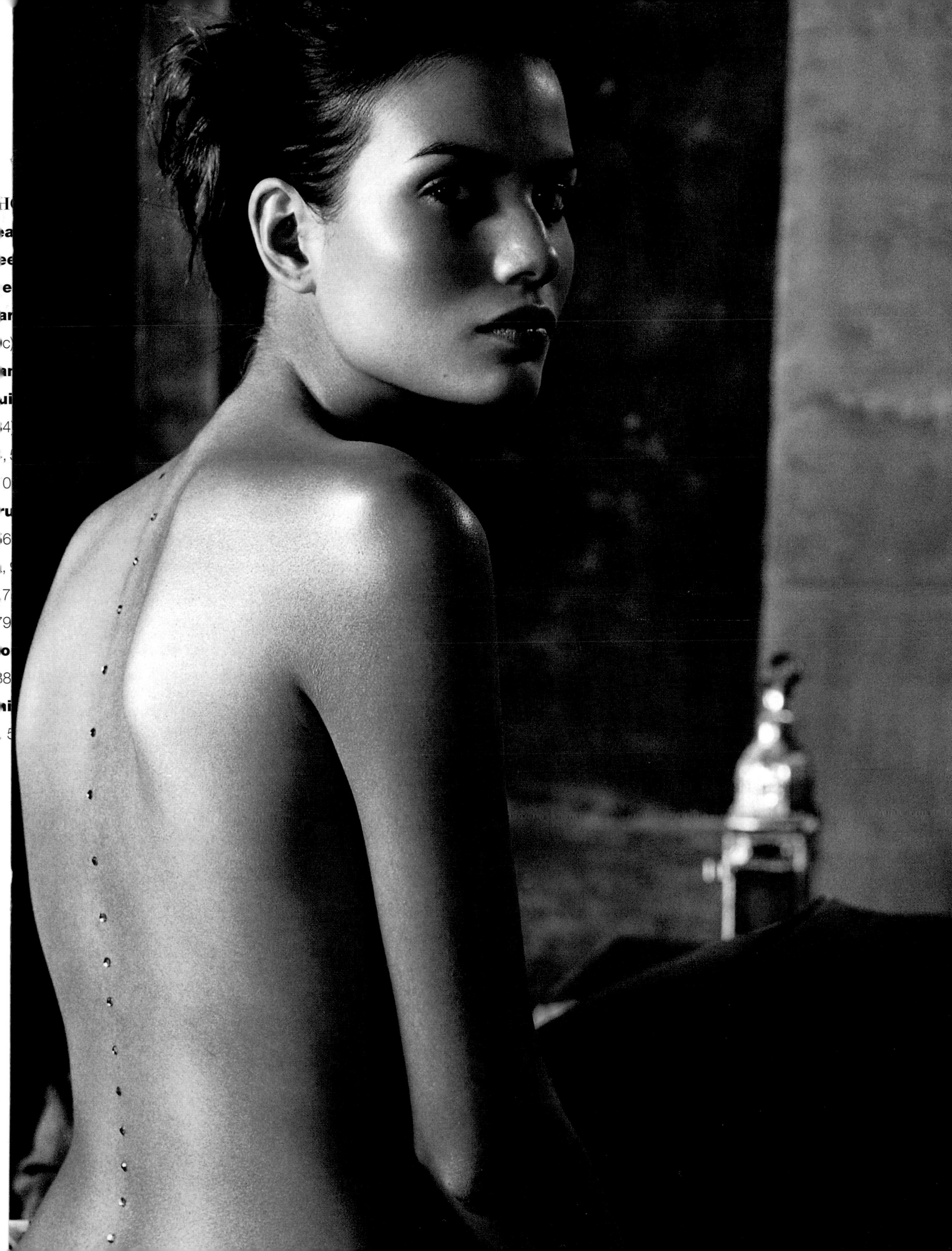

Original title: FACE & BODY

www.marieclairebooks.com

General Director, Marie Claire Album SA: Arnaud de Contades
President, Marie Claire Album SA: Évelyne Prousost-Berry

Editorial Director: Thierry Lamarre
Concept, Interviews, and Editing: Josette Milgram
English Translation: Kim Allen Gleed
Layout editing: Nicolas Valoteau
Assistant editor: Julie Bavant
Editorial assistant: Adeline Lobut
Artwork and design: Domitille Peyron, SylvieCreusy, Marie Niogret

Library of Congress Cataloging-in-Publication Data is available for this title.

10 9 8 7 6 5 4 3 2 1

PUBLISHED BY HEARST BOOKS
A Division of Sterling Publishing Co., Inc.
387 Park Avenue South, New York, NY 10016

www.marieclaire.com

Distributed in Canada by Sterling Publishing
c/o Canadian Manda Group, 165 Dufferin Street
Toronto, Ontario, Canada M6K 3H6

For information about custom editions, special sales, premium and corporate purchases, please contact Sterling Special Sales Department at 800-805-5489 or specialsales@sterlingpublishing.com.

Manufactured in China

Sterling ISBN: 978-1-58816-667-8